Think and Grow Rich in Dentistry

Published by CelebrityPress®, Orlando, FL

CelebrityPress® is a registered trademark.

Printed in the United States of America.

ISBN: 978-0-9966887-2-7
LCCN: 2015946669

This publication is designed to provide accurate and authoritative information with regard to the subject matter covered. It is sold with the understanding that the publisher is not engaged in rendering legal, accounting, or other professional advice. If legal advice or other expert assistance is required, the services of a competent professional should be sought. The opinions expressed by the authors in this book are not endorsed by CelebrityPress® and are the sole responsibility of the author rendering the opinion.

Most CelebrityPress® titles are available at special quantity discounts for bulk purchases for sales promotions, premiums, fundraising, and educational use. Special versions or book excerpts can also be created to fit specific needs.

For more information, please write:
CelebrityPress®
520 N. Orlando Ave, #2
Winter Park, FL 32789
or call 1.877.261.4930

Visit us online at: www.CelebrityPressPublishing.com

Think and Grow Rich in Dentistry

55 Time-Tested Principles For Success

By

Steven K. Brown

CelebrityPress®

Winter Park, Florida

Author's Preface

HELLO, my name is Kelly Brown. I graduated from the University of Oklahoma College of Dentistry in 1976. Like the majority of my classmates upon graduating, I moved to my preferred community, threw out a shingle, hired a couple of folks and opened my practice. Although this formula at the time didn't provide me with a successful practice, I did stay out of bankruptcy court, jail and lawsuits, which would surely be the results today.

Over the last 36 years, dentistry, government regulations, employees and patients have all drastically changed. Naivety today comes with a very expensive price tag. One most dentists don't need to pay.

Over the years I have trained, mentored, associated and partnered with well over 100 dentists. I have birthed more solo dental practices than any other dentist in the world. It is my intent with this book to guide you around the pitfalls of going into private practice, save you time and money.

I hope you use my experience and knowledge to build your wisdom and become a productive, profitable dental practitioner.

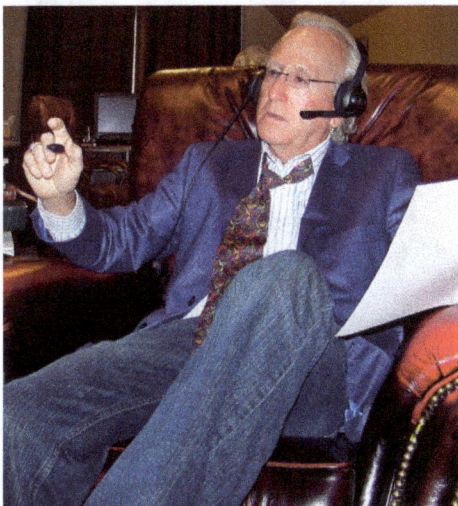

Acknowledgements

Writing a book is much like giving birth. Once the seed is planted there are many arduous months of labor before the book is born. There have been many important patient people helping me through the labor pains.

First, I must thank, Jan, my wife for having the patience of spending many valuable vacation hours with me chasing down the roots of Dr. Edgar Parker. She also tolerated my many hours locked away in my man cave pounding on these keys.

Next I would like to thank Evelyn Ferchau and my Marketing Coordinator, Teri Hirlinger for shouldering the painful task of word-smithing and formatting this book. Although I knew in my heart what I wanted to deliver, without these women, I'm afraid you wouldn't have been able to read it.

I would also like to thank Scott Parman, Robert Echols, Dr James Stocker and Dr. Chris Griffin for taking the time to read and critique this book in its early stages.

Nothing worth value is truly created without a great team and my baby, Think and Grow Rich in Dentistry, had the best.

To

My Wife and Best Friend, Jan

Table of Contents

Chapter One

INTRODUCTION

*"A successful man is one who can lay a firm foundation
with the bricks others have thrown at him."*

DAVID BRINKLEY

MY father was a J.C. Penney's manager; my mother was a housewife. Our home was always full of love, yet empty of cash. The words "We can't afford that" were used more frequently than the vacuum cleaner.

I remember one day when I was about 12 having a conversation with my mom that went like this, *"Mom, when I grow up, I'm going to be rich. I'm not sure how and I hope it's legal."*

The words of advice dispensed by my parents and teachers were *"If you want to get ahead in life, you need a good education."* That meant, of course, going to college.

So in 1969 I headed off to Norman and the University of Oklahoma in hopes of finding my fortune. It wasn't long before I discovered none of my college professors were rich. How were they going to pass me the keys to the vault when their key rings were empty?

My hope was revived when I was accepted into dental school. But it flickered a short while when I discovered that a dental diploma didn't guarantee you passage into the elite club of folks who have more passive income than they will ever spend.

This is when I started searching for those who knew how to escape "The Rat Race," as wealth coach Robert Kiyosaki calls it, and move to the "Fast Track."

I remember going to the book store with my wife, Jan, one day. While she was looking for a book, I noticed a section in the store titled "Business and Personal Development." There were volumes of books on making money: how to become rich as an inventor; how to get rich in real estate; how to get rich selling things out of your home; etc. All of these looked good to me... except I was in dental school. I didn't have much time, and I had absolutely no money. Then I saw it—Think and Grow Rich by Napolean Hill. Now, I could do that. If all I needed to do was "think" and I could become rich, count me in.

Over the years I have read Think and Grow Rich many times. It has always been inspiring, but sometimes I had trouble applying the principles to my practice.

Think and Grow Rich in Dentistry is my attempt to put dental meat on the principles of Think and Grow Rich by telling the stories of two dentists, Dr. Edgar Randolph Rudolph Parker, aka "Painless Parker," and myself. This book is full of real-life issues dentists face every day and situational decisions that make a difference.

For those looking for a path from the "Rat Race" to the "Fast Track" using the profession of dentistry, buying this book and consuming its content will provide you the keys to the vault that will liberate you and reward your family.

Chapter Two

A THREE-DOG LIFE

"You have to learn the rules of the game. And then you have to play better than anyone else."

ALBERT EINSTEIN

WHAT I'm about to share with you can have a profound effect on your life and business. It can boost your results, turn prospects into patients and, ultimately, give you the success and income you want. In the balance of this book I will explain more, but in the meantime, let's travel back to 1976.

The month was October. That January the Pittsburg Steelers beat the Dallas Cowboys in Super Bowl X, Jimmy Carter was running for president, the Cray-1 released the first commercially developed super computer and composite was a questionable new material. There were no light cured composites, intra-oral cameras, digital x-rays or even dental computers to be found for decades to come. Root canals took three, one-hour appointments and porcelain fused to metal was on the cutting edge of cosmetic dentistry. A dental office could be built and equipped for $50,000 and a 24-year-old boy/man saw his first private practice patient.

To camouflage my youth, I sported a full beard to compliment my shoulder-length hair. My first 60-year-old female patient loudly questioned the assistant when I left the room. *"Nurse. Nurse! Was that my dentist?"*

Back in the 60s one of my favorite bands was "Three Dog Night." Little did I know I was in for a Three-Dog Life. The first dog was a playful pup, only interested in girls and getting through school with as little effort as possible, in that order. God had His hand on me when I met Jan Gates. Looking back 42 years, we are both confused at what attracted her to me. She says somewhere under that long hair and deep in those marijuana glazed eyes, she saw potential.

I'm not sure if it is a strength or a weakness, but my insatiable desire to please, in this case, Jan flung me head long into a course that would ultimately take me to dental school. I would like to say the years with Jan and finishing dental school made me a better person, but that was not the case.

By 1987 (11 years into practice if you are math challenged), I found myself in a solo practice in my hometown of Guthrie, Oklahoma, with two sons and an overly supportive wife. My practice was full of unhappy patients. My staff was miserable and my bank account was anemic. Past due bills and overloaded credit cards were the only things to be found in abundance.

The second-dog life was a bull dog. I remember the day just like it was yesterday. It was June 25, 1987. I remember walking into my office after the worst week of my life. I had just buried my two-year-old son who had died in a tragic accident. I was feeling the pain of that and the embarrassment of having to pay for his burial with yet another credit card. I had been out of the office for a week and I knew I would be facing a schedule full of folks who were half ticked, plus a pile of unopened mail.

Well, that day on top of the stack of mail found on my small, cluttered desk was a 3 x 5 yellow card. I am sure it had been in my mail many times before, but in my busyness it was perceived as pesky junk mail. That day, however, I picked it up and read it. It was pure and simple and spoke straight to my pain. It said "Doctor, Have You Had Enough? Is It Time You Take Control of Your Life? Call This Number for A Free Consultation." I closed the door to my tiny office, sat down at my messy desk and made a call that would change my life. That day the post card, once perceived as a pest, became a welcome guest.

The person who answered my desperate call was good. He asked the right questions, was empathetic with my pain and even though I didn't want to hear it, told me exactly what I needed to do next. He said *"Doctor, we can help, however you will need to be in Glendale, California, for a training program next week."*

Mark Twain said, *"There are basically two kinds of folks, those with excuses and those with results."* If I was looking for excuses that day, I had a few to pick from. I had just buried my son. I had been out of the office for a week already. Nathan, my surviving son, and my wife needed me at home for emotional support. I would need another credit card. These were just a few. However, that day I was not looking for excuses, I was looking for relief from my pain. So, I applied for another credit card, told my bewildered receptionist that I was taking off for another week, kissed my son and wife good bye and the bull dog headed off to Glendale for a journey that brings me here today.

My third-dog life is a Saint Bernard. After hundreds of hours in classes, stacks of continuing education cassettes (this dates me) and a six-figure business education investment, I was able to take my fledgling dental practice from the bottom of the heap to the top 1%-producing solo practices in the U.S. I then became the Saint Bernard, rescuing dentists from the same practice perils I knew so well.

Over the years I have been invited to be a guest speaker in several diverse venues. Although I was fortunate to share the stage with many prestigious pros like Zig Ziglar, John Maxwell and Roger Staubach, my favorite audiences were dental students. I still get invited to speak on dental management to junior and senior students. And I enjoy it immensely. Being thrust back into the academic environment, I learned something distressful. For various reasons, the dental manpower in the rural communities was trending downward. Very few new graduates have the financial resources and the professional confidence to venture out to these communities and set up a practice.

In the Oklahoma rural market there were more dentists dying or retiring than new graduates willing to replace them. In 2001, I had a long-time friend and colleague approach me about working in my office after he had fulfilled his service obligation with the Indian Health Service. I was hesitant because over the years I had tried and failed miserably to incorporate an associate into my practice. Not wanting to say no, I had another idea. By this time I had developed a very successful practice with many proprietary systems. Could I help my friend duplicate my success in another location?

In July of 2002, we launched what was to become the second Custom Dental practice. Today Custom Dental has replicated itself 10 times in Missouri and Oklahoma and we have plans to add many more. This unique operating model allows dentists to be in business for themselves, but not by themselves. In 2008, I left my chair-side practice to support and mentor my partner docs as Custom Dental became the fastest growing owner-operated joint venture dental business in the world.

I share my story with you to let you know your guide on this tour didn't fall off the turnip truck yesterday. If you are struggling, I know your pain. If you already have a good practice but want more, I understand and admire your ambition.

So now, allow me to be your guide.

Chapter Three

THE SECRETS FOR YOUR FUTURE SUCCESS ARE HIDDEN IN THE PAST

"You can't connect the dots looking forward; you can only connect them looking backwards. So you have to trust that the dots will somehow connect in your future. You have to trust in something – your gut, destiny, life, karma, whatever. This approach has never let me down, and it has made all the difference in my life."

STEVE JOBS

THE square was bustling with noise. People with cameras were scurrying to the next location. Masses of humanity with headphones gathered in groups around someone explaining what they were witnessing. Others were aimlessly wandering through the ancient public square, glancing down at a booklet or folded paper with a look of total confusion.

My wife and I and another couple were traveling in Italy and had decided to hire a private guide in Venice. She was an attractive 32-year-old Venetian girl. She spoke very good English, although it came across with a slight local accent.

At this moment she had gathered the four of us into a secluded area of the Piazza San Marco Square away from the noise, to explain what I recall to be a most incredible, eye-opening phenomenon.

As we stood in the north side of the Piazza San Marco staring at St. Mark's Clocktower, the guide began to describe this incredible blue-faced, gold-highlighted 12-foot diameter clock, located half way up the ornate 50-foot tower. This magnificent mechanical device was more complicated than the watch I was wearing, was built over

500 years earlier and was still working perfectly. The majestic clock face was blue with gold inside a fixed circle of marble, which was engraved with the 24 hours of the day in Roman numerals. A golden pointer with an image of the sun moved around the circle, indicating the hour of the day. Within the marble circle beneath the sun pointer were the signs of the zodiac in gold, revolving slightly more slowly than the pointer to show the position of the sun in the zodiac. The earth took center position in the middle of the clock face as the moon revolved around the earth to show its phases, surrounded by stars fixed in position.

What was fascinating about this complex piece of work was that while the seconds, minutes, hours, days and months passed, the perpetual motion, internal mechanism positioned each symbol in perfect harmony to the correct time, zodiac symbol and earth-moon positioning. And it had for over 500 years.

My mind started to drift as our guide redirected our attention to the Saint Mark's Basilica just to the right of the tower. Five hundred years and still working? How could this intricate clock be created without modern day technology? What was the clock builder's secret?

Much like that busy Italian square, our industry is bustling with dentists gathered in groups to hear about the next shiny object that promises to flood their offices with new patients begging for care. I contend that all this confusion and noise has hidden the age-old truths on how to succeed in dentistry. So for the rest of this book, allow me to be your tour guide, pull you out of the crowd and, with my local accent, disclose the principles of practice success through the life of a dentist, Edgar Randolph Rudolph Parker, aka "Painless Parker," who over a century ago built a dental empire that has yet to be matched.

Chapter Four

WHO IS PAINLESS PARKER?

"Here's to the crazy ones. The misfits. The rebels. The troublemakers. The round pegs in the square holes. The ones who see things differently. They're not fond of rules. And they have no respect for the status quo. You can quote them, disagree with them, glorify or vilify them. About the only thing you can't do is ignore them. Because they change things. They push the human race forward. And while some may see them as the crazy ones, we see genius. Because the people who are crazy enough to think they can change the world, are the ones who do."

STEVE JOBS

SO why do I consider Edgar Randolph Rudolph Parker, later known as "Painless Parker," a dental icon? Although he has been dead for over 60 years, the name of Painless Parker can still evoke amongst some dentists unpleasant emotions and a stereotyped image of dentistry at its worst. However, the true story of this man not only reveals he was larger than life but his ideas and principles are still found driving some of the most successful dental practices. Employing these principles Parker racked up a long list of intriguing accomplishments.

By 1900, at the age of 26, only two years after arriving in Brooklyn, Parker had built 17 Parker clinics throughout the New York City area and was generating what would be in today's money about $100M per year. One of the 17 offices housed 15 dentists with 45 chairs.

In 1906, at the age of 34, he sold all his Brooklyn area holdings and retired to Los Angeles, California. After a few short months of rest, Parker just couldn't stay out of the dental game. When presented an opportunity to start all over in California, he took it. Within two months, he had established four dental offices that were generating in today's economy a $100K per day. By 1910 he had built a dental business that dwarfed his first New York empire.

In 1915, when the state of California passed state statute No. 426, which compelled dentists to practice under their legal names, Edgar Randolph Rudolph Parker legally changed his first name to "Painless." He went on to develop Painless Parker dental products and founded the Parker Institute of Dental Economics where he trained dental graduates, technicians and assistants in the E.R. Parker systems of dental delivery. At the time of his death in 1952, Painless still had 28 dental offices spread up and down the west coast.

His renegade attitude helped shape the American Dental Association and many state dental regulatory bodies.

How did a man with such humble beginnings make such an impact on the dental profession? How could he, seemingly at will, create a demand for dental care, and then provide it?

It is my intention to peel back the onion on Painless Parker's life and reveal these principles to you. And if you are open-minded and maybe even bold enough, you may find yourself implementing a few of them. So let's start with how I ran across Painless Parker.

Chapter Five

HOW I MET PAINLESS

"The difference between a successful person and others is not a lack of strength, not a lack of knowledge, but rather a lack of will."

VINCE LOMBARDI

Although Painless Parker died in 1952, a year after my birth, his legend still lived on with many of my dental professors, particularly those who graduated from USC. The first time I heard his name it was not very complimentary. You must remember back in 1976 the prevailing attitude about advertising dentists could be compared to that of a pole dancer, with Painless Parker being the feature attraction.

After dental school, I didn't hear much about him. It wasn't until 2011, when I was doing some marketing research that I ran across an author named Dr. Arden G. Christen. Along with many other publications, Dr. Christen had edited one book on Painless Parker, The Early Adventures of Painless Parker, and authored Painless Parker: A Dental Renegade's Fight to Make Advertising Ethical.

On Amazon I found The Early Adventures of Painless Parker. There were only two copies available. They were both used and cost over $100 each. My first thought was, *"Wow, a used paperback for over $100. You've got to be kidding me. Maybe I don't need this old book that bad."* However, my curiosity got the best of me and I placed the order.

Unfortunately, the book never reached me. I had forgotten to change my Amazon profile to reflect a recent address change. The book was actually sold by an Amazon affiliate; therefore I got no cooperation on locating it. I checked Amazon today and there are two books available starting at, get this, $1,396.27 each. Ouch.

I was a little perturbed but still determined to get the book, so I did a search for the author, Arden G. Christen. Although getting up in years, I found he was still alive and teaching at Indiana School of Dentistry.

I paid an online service to find his address. When I got it, I wrote him a letter expressing my desire for The Early Adventures of Painless Parker and Painless Parker, A Dental Renegade's Fight to Make Advertising Ethical.

It was a long shot that paid off. A few weeks later I received a very nice handwritten note from Dr. Christen telling me that if I would send him $20 for each book, he would mail them to me. I immediately followed those instructions and within two weeks, I was the proud owner of both.

After reading both books multiple times, I would have to say if I had paid the $1,396.27 it would have still been a bargain. I was so fascinated by Parker's story and his insights into timeless principles that I decided to go back and visit his roots on my next summer vacation.

On July 26, 2012, Jan and I headed to Halifax by air and rented a car to explore the Bay of Fundy and the stomping grounds of young Painless Parker. Come with me as I begin to highlight my trip, Parker's childhood experiences and how they impacted this dental legend.

Chapter Six

EXPLORING PARKER'S ROOTS

"Desire is the key to motivation, but it's determination and commitment to an unrelenting pursuit of your goal - a commitment to excellence - that will enable you to attain the success you seek."

MARIO ANDRETTI

After a few days in Halifax and an evening in Moncton, New Brunswick, I greatly anticipated the next morning when we would finally visit Tynemouth Creek, New Brunswick, Parker's birthplace. First we headed south until reaching the Bay of Fundy. We stopped along the way to admire the unique tide patterns. In some coastal areas on this bay, the difference between low and high tide is over 50 feet. This tide phenomenon is caused by the shape of the bay. It has a very large ocean entrance and constricts as it moves toward the coast. Our park guide explained that it is like forcing water into a corner of a bathtub.

As we left this area we continued westward following the coastline down long and windy roads, passing through tiny fishing villages. My wife and I were starving by this time and felt like sailors lost at sea, dying of thirst. Lobster farms were abundant, but there was no place to eat.

After studying the map we determined the first town of any Parker significance would be St. Martins. St. Martins was once an

PRINCIPLE 1

Determination is the key to all success.

important ship-building center but today it is a town village with a population of 380, 40 kilometers east of Saint John. It is located on the shores of the famous Bay of Fundy. St. Martins is a beautiful, picturesque settlement with a rich history. The scenic village has many interesting features, including Victorian properties; miles of unspoiled, quiet, accessible beaches; two lighthouses; a garden-park; an active harbor boasting two covered bridges; world famous "Sea Caves" and the title of "The Gateway to the Fundy Trail."

We stopped at one of the lighthouses to stretch our legs, research our dining prospects and, hopefully, find some proud local Painless Parker fans. Stretching was all that was accomplished on this stop.

I will soon disclose how St. Martins played a very important role in developing our hero, but first, we again loaded up in the car and continued 14 kilometers westward towards St. John. There we ran into an even smaller coastal community, Tynemouth Creek, New Brunswick, Canada. And there is where it all began.

Go back with me to 1875. The U.S. population had just reached 50 million, while the sparsely populated Canada was approaching 4 million. George F. Green had patented the dental drill. Alexander Graham Bell and his assistant had discovered that sound could be transported by wire. In 1878 Woolworth opened what he called a "five- and ten-cent store." And in 1884 a surgeon named Dr. William Stewart Halsted developed a highly successful local anesthetic technique using cocaine.

PRINCIPLE 2

Public speaking can be a powerful tool.

All of these occurrences were preceded by the birth of someone who would eventually revolutionize the dental world, Edgar Randolph Rudolph Parker. On Friday, March 22, 1872, at five A.M., this dental icon was born on the bleak and rocky shores of the Bay of Fundy. He was the eldest of six born to George and Jennie Parker, and one of four boys to survive the harsh and unforgiving environment.

George owned a shipbuilding yard in Tynemouth Creek, which would eventually fail in 1884. This forced the family to move to a small town, St. Martins, seven miles northeast where George bought a livery stable.

Let's take a break here to explore a few important episodes in Parker's early years. These taught him important principles that would eventually catapult him into a league of his own.

When Parker was six he attended a one-room school in Tynemouth Creek. He was quite smitten with his 18-year-old teacher, Mary Bradshaw. She had blues eyes and light fluffy blond hair. She was second only to his mother in his adoration. When it was time for Edgar to learn his ABCs, he thoroughly enjoyed her attention.

One day Edgar was asked to stand in front of the class and recite the alphabet to his giggly, fidgeting group of classmates. After about four or five letters, he could go no further. He was so embarrassed and upset that he had let Miss Bradshaw down that he dropped his head and slipped quietly back into his seat. Although the experience was quite disappointing to all, Edgar was determined to learn his alphabet. He grit his teeth, pursed his lips and pored intently over the pages of his primer, which contained the alphabet printed in large, bold letters.

No matter how hard he tried, every time Edgar got up to recite his ABCs, he invariably got stuck less than half the way through and had to sit down, more embarrassed but still more determined than before.

PRINCIPLE 3

The key to success is differentiation.

"Differentiate or Die."

It had become such an obstacle that Edgar confided in his mom about his difficulty. Greatly concerned with her son's ability to master the very rudiments of learning and language, Jennie Parker took it upon herself to help him conquer his learning block. Try as she would, she couldn't get any better results than Miss Bradshaw.

Finally, in desperation, she broke down in tears. Edgar could hear between his mother's sobs, her bemoaning the fact of having such a stupid son. Edgar was doubly devastated: he had obviously disappointed both of the most important people in his life.

He had to quickly think of a reasonable explanation to regain their favor and approval.

Suddenly a bright smile came over his face, and with great composure he spoke up. *"Mother, he blurted out, "I know the alphabet, all right. I can read the primer as good as anyone in my class, but I still can't say the alphabet the way you and Miss Bradshaw want me to."*

His mother looked bewildered.

"What do you mean?" she asked, somewhat perplexed. *"Just how do you prefer to recite the alphabet?"*

"This way," he replied cheerfully, *"Z, X, W, V, U, T, S, R, Q, P, O, N, M, L, K, J, I, H, G, F, E, D, C, B, A."* No one knew exactly how he could do this, but today we call it dyslexia.

His mother was astounded. She went to school with Edgar the next morning to show Miss Bradshaw.

Miss Bradshaw's tinkling laughter echoed throughout the schoolroom, and the other pupils who had overheard the conversation between teacher and parent, cheered and clapped.

Edgar's determination had paid off. He learned how to struggle through difficulties and became a great public speaker. He also learned that if you can do it different than everyone else, you will always get more attention.

Even though it was a battle, Edgar became excellent at the alphabet. Overcoming with determination became his creed and a lifestyle that would eventually separate him from his peers.

I was accepted to dental school at the age of 20. My only experience in a dental office was at the wrong end of a drill. Everything about dental school was absolutely foreign to me. I was always the last to finish all the pre-clinical exercises and clinical procedures. While grading my attempts my professors would make demeaning comments like, *"Did you really do this with your hands?"*

By the time I had graduated, I had developed a good case of inferiority. I spent the first five years of my practice struggling clinically. But I forced myself into situations where I could watch those more proficient than myself. Eventually, I started to believe I could get better, and I did. By the time I had retired from patient care, I could keep up with the best.

My financial development followed a similar pattern. I came

from a family rich with love but bankrupt in the language of money. As I have mentioned earlier, I was a financial disaster well into my dental career. But in 1987, I decided to break my genetic chains and escape monetary pressures. I read every book I could get my hands on, went to numerous seminars and filled my car with cassettes on the topic. Within 10 years, I had gotten my financial house in order. So much so that today I enjoy a life not dictated by the lack of money.

Just because you are not good at something, doesn't mean you have to stay there. In dentistry, and in business, you must personally overcome your shortcomings through determination, or be determined to find someone on your team to fill in the gap.

Even though his first attempt at public speaking was a total flop Parker continued to try until he succeeded. He eventually turned this initial weakness into a great success.

My mom thought that it was cute for her children to be on the plump side, so by the fourth grade I was 4'7" tall and weighed 105 pounds. I was always the short fat one, front and center, in all my grade school pictures. The thought of standing in front of people, much less speaking made me want to vomit. I fought this phobia until 1979. At that time I had joined a network marketing business. For those who don't know, this is a business primarily geared around recruiting teams of people to sell merchandise. Remember, I am starving on my dental income at this time, so I became intrigued with any opportunity to make more money.

One night, while in the back of the room watching a group business opportunity presentation, I realized the only guy in the room making money was the one in front presenting the plan. At that moment I decided to overcome my fear and learn how to deliver the marketing message to groups.

My first victim was Ralph, our two-year-old basset hound. I propped him up on the couch, got out my white board and delivered my first public speech. After I had finally practiced enough with Ralph I decided to give it a shot with a few friends and neighbors. Eventually, I was presenting the plan in hotel rooms with over 100 attendees. That grew into stadiums full of people. I even made a presentation in Germany in front of 4,000 attendees with interpreters from six countries. Kelly Brown had traversed a long path from the pudgy, shy fourth grader.

If I hadn't forced myself to start with Ralph, I would have never had the courage to speak in front of dental classes, which ultimately lead me to the development of Custom Dental.

It is said public speaking is feared more than death itself by the majority of the population. This is an even bigger reason why developing those skills is important. When you have the courage to address a group, you automatically move up in their minds. The most successful people I know in any profession have developed the skill of communication. There are books, CDs, DVDs and courses on developing this skill.

Public speaking can be an opportunity to success or a stumbling block leading to failure. It is a skill and can be learned. How would you rate yourself in this principle?

Although Edgar could eventually recite his alphabet anyway he wanted, he realized when he did it differently he received more attention. He would eventually use this principle to build a dental empire. I did the same.

I started using the differentiation principle in 1987. I was the first dentist in my community to use direct mail, erect aggressive signage, be featured on a local TV news broadcast, write a book, offer implants, etc. The list goes on.

I wake up every morning and ask myself these questions, *"What can I say that Custom Dental does differently than anyone else? Why should my public give me and my partners special attention?"*

If you can answer these questions with a clear and concise answer, you are well on your way. If you can't, you need to spend some time here until you can.

Chapter Seven

EDGAR'S FIRST BUSINESS

"Develop success from failures. Discouragement and failure are two of the surest stepping stones to success."

DALE CARNEGIE

When Edgar was about nine years old, he and his six-year-old sister, Bessie, decided to become chicken farmers. The previous year Edgar and Bessie had walked 10 miles round trip to school every day and developed a close sibling tie. Early in May as school was wrapping up, they had heard of an old lady, Mrs. Fraser, in the village who wanted to sell a setting Plymouth Rock hen, complete with hen coop and 13 eggs. The rumor had it that Mrs. Fraser did not feel well and couldn't take care of the little chicks that she was expecting from the setting hen.

Edgar excitedly talked it over with Bessie. With visions of becoming bona fide chicken farmers filling their minds and stirring their imaginations, they began to contrive ways to obtain that setting hen and her eggs.

Mrs. Fraser lived alone in a snug cottage tucked in a clearing nestled in the woods. She was short, plump and had round, rosy cheeks. Although Mrs. Fraser didn't look ill, she told Edgar and Bessie that her rheumatism made it difficult for her to get around.

PRINCIPLE 4

You can only succeed if you try.

She wanted 40 cents for the hen, the eggs and the coop. She

took them out to a shed to show them the setup. The coop turned out to be a rusty, oval stove made of sheet metal.

After seeing the hen and eggs and quickly assessing the possibilities, Edgar wanted that hen and setting of eggs more than anything else in the world. With that incentive, he gave Mrs. Fraser the first of what would become many sales pitches. (Who would have predicted this nine-year-old boy becoming the master salesmen of all times?)

Edgar told her that they didn't have any money, but since they were children of George Sancton Parker, who lived at the mouth of Tynemouth Creek, they could be trusted. Furthermore, if she let them have the hen and eggs, they could easily retire the debt from the money they would earn by selling cranberries and eggs to the fishermen and sailors later that year. (This was also the first of many no-money-down business deals Edgar would attempt.)

Mrs. Fraser didn't buy it. The entire process would take too long.

Edgar's young but keen business mind now went into a state of hyper activity. He thought of the fish they could catch in the pools in Tynemouth Creek harbor. They were left there when the tides went out. So he asked Mrs. Fraser if they could barter fresh fish for the hen and eggs.

Quite abruptly, Mrs. Fraser brightened. These children had a good idea.

"I like fresh fish," she said. *"Do you know how to clean them?"*

"Yes, Ma'am," Edgar replied proudly.

"Alright, alright," she said, *"Seeing as you are George and Jennie Parker's children, I know you will keep your word. Do you want to take the hen now?"*

PRINCIPLE 5

If you can find out what people want, you can have anything you want.

"Yes!" both Edgar and Bessie piped up.

It was a nearly two-mile hike back to their home. Bessie grabbed the front legs of the stove and Edgar the back legs and off they went with hen, eggs and coop in tow. They had the beginnings of their first business, a chicken farm.

At first, everything went fine. They were so happy and proud of their achievement; they seemed to effortlessly carry the prized acqui-

PRINCIPLE 6
It is never as easy as it seems at first.

sition homeward. But eventually the initial burst of adrenaline wore off and Bessie began to gasp for air. The coop suddenly seemed very heavy. Bessie and Edgar set the hen coop, hen and eggs gingerly down on a stump to rest. Just how many times they would repeat that same routine before arriving home is uncertain.

Because it was early spring and the snow was melting, their path was rough and muddy in spots. The mother hen was severely shaken up during the moving ordeal, but refused to leave her nest and eggs. Occasionally she would let out a few frightened squawks when the children would slip and slide in the mud, but she never flew out even though the stove had no lid.

When Edgar and Bessie finally got their prize acquisition home, it was long after dark and supper time. As you could imagine, their parents were beside themselves. What could have happened to a nine- and six-year-old in the wilderness around Tynemouth Creek?

PRINCIPLE 7
Always make good on your debt.

Although their mom had a few guarded words of approval for their new business acquisition, their dad responded with "Kids' foolishness."

Although the next day was Saturday and Edgar was out of school, he woke early ready to make good on his debt.

When he glanced out the window, he saw the tide ebbing fast so that the harbor would soon be empty. He roused Bessie, reminding her of the seriousness of their financial obligation. He told her that she needed to help him catch some fish.

Bessie dressed in a jiffy and they headed out to the harbor bottom now exposed due to the low tide. They hunted together, wading through the sticky red, gooey mud and the tide pools, searching for their prize.

Bessie screamed when she found a pool with a fiddler salmon. It was a young and healthy fish of good size.

PRINCIPLE 8

Don't expect everyone around you to understand.

Their next problem would be retrieving the squirming catch and getting it to Mrs. Fraser to reduce their debt.

Edgar reached down and stroked the fish on the back to see what might happen. Nothing happened! The salmon didn't seem to mind. As a matter of fact it seemed to move closer to Edgar's side of the pool. Edgar repeated the process and the salmon continued to move closer, as though it liked it and wanted more. Eventually the docile fish lay over against the edge of the pool exposing its whole silvery length. Edgar's temptation was to make a pet out of the fish, but the thought of his debt would not allow him the pleasure. So, he gritted his teeth, put one hand just behind the salmon's gills and another under its rudder-like tail, and, with a sudden, tremendous heave, flipped the sedate fish bodily out of the water and onto the muddy harbor bottom.

The fiddler salmon came alive immediately. It flopped out of Edgar's hands and fought with astonishing strength. Edgar and the salmon proceeded to wrestle; each knowing what was at stake. As the battle progressed, the only thing on Edgar that was not totally covered in the red sticky mud was his eyes. After what seemed to be a lifetime for all involved, out of sheer exhaustion the salmon finally gave up. It had been a good fight, but Edgar's determination had finally paid off!

When Edgar and Bessie eventually got the fish to shore, they weighed him. The salmon tipped the scale at 14 pounds and was two feet long.

During the struggle Edgar had developed a weird respect for the magnificent fish and with a sense of remorse of killing such a "pet;" he cleaned and prepared the salmon.

Immediately after preparing the salmon Bessie and Edgar set off to deliver their catch to Mrs. Fraser, believing this payment to be a good installment on their debt.

Fresh salmon at that time of the year was considered a great delicacy. So, when the children lifted the cover off the basket and revealed the nicely prepared deep-sea fiddler salmon, plump Mrs. Fraser fairly squealed with delight. *"Oh, you wonderful children!"* she exclaimed. *"That is one of the nicest salmon I have ever seen!"*

She lifted the salmon out of the basket, nearly hugging it. She put it on a platter and then asked, *"Isn't that dulce in that basket?"* (Dulce is edible seaweed that was prized by the locals.)

"Yes, Ma'am," the children answered in unison. *"Oh, I love dulce,"* said Mrs. Fraser, *"Why don't you children gather more of it, dry it and sell it to the people on the farms hereabouts? Only you folks who live right on the bay can have all you want."*

The children thanked her for the suggestion, but at the moment Edgar's big worry was paying off their debt. He drew in his breath, mustered up his courage and asked, *"How many more fish do we have to bring to you before we eliminate our debt?"*

"Oh you've paid your debt already," replied Mrs. Fraser. *"That gorgeous salmon is worth every bit as much as the hen and the settings of eggs, and the dulce is worth something, too. You can consider your debt paid off in full, with interest."*

Edgar couldn't have been happier. He had borrowed money to start a business and had already paid it back. The weight of the world was off his back.

Edgar's father was quite skeptical of the children's ability to succeed at business. This made Edgar even more determined.

That summer was quite lucrative for Edgar and Bessie. They sold fish, dulce, frying chickens and eggs to the sailors and fishermen. With the cash they made, they would buy tobacco, clay pipes and many other consumer items in St. Martins. Then they sold them back in Tynemouth Creek to residents who had requested such items. Edgar had learned five more success principles and had taken his first step into entrepreneurship. It would carry him through for the next seven decades.

There were three frogs on a log. Two decided to jump off. How many frogs are left? If you answered *"one,"* you are wrong. There are still three frogs on the log until a frog actually does more than decides to jump off. As the distance between deciding and doing is expanded, the likelihood of doing diminishes.

You can sometimes analyze an opportunity until you become paralyzed. Although Edgar was only nine years old, and had no previous business experience or money, he still decided to go into the chicken business. He wasn't afraid to take immediate action to make that happen.

Upon returning from my first of many management seminars in June, 1987, I plunged headfirst into implementing the strategies and systems I had learned. If you think my great revelation was appreciated by my staff at that time, you are wrong.

It was like pushing hot molasses up a flag pole. I was confronted by my staff with, *"That will never work in a dental practice. That will never work in our town. Why should we change? We have never done it that way before."*

The bad news is I ultimately lost all but one staff member within the next four weeks. The good news is I eventually replaced them with a team I still enjoy working with today.

Looking back I am convinced that had I thought and worried about how I was going to become a businessman who could transition my sick practice into a prize gem, I would still be worrying today.

What additional services, community outreach programs or business modifications would improve your practice? How many of your good ideas have died an untimely death because you wanted to wait until all the stars lined up and the time was perfect?

Robert Echols, a bootstrap multi-millionaire and friend of mine says, *"You can't steer a parked car." Will you make mistakes and face some failures? Absolutely! If you don't, it wouldn't be fair to the rest of us who have. Remember this: "The road to success is paved with well managed mistakes."* Leadership guru and author John Maxwell, calls it "Failing Forward."

Many times we build, buy or create a product or service, then try to find people who want it. In this story, Edgar found out what Mrs. Fraser wanted and started his venture. He later used the same technique to expand his business to sailors, fishermen and other local people.

A very successful restaurant owner was asked what the most important asset in his business was and he replied, *"A hungry crowd."*

Many dentists try to sell crowns, braces, root canals and implants. That is a huge mistake. Patients don't want any of those things. They want comfort and confidence. A good question for you is "What are you selling in your office?"

Acquiring Mrs. Fraser's hen, eggs and coop seemed like a simple task to begin with. But Edgar and Bessie soon found out it was a struggle to complete the total transaction. Several times they almost fell and lost the entire opportunity.

As I made mention of earlier, from 1987 to 2001 I had tried several associateship and partner models in my office. All of which miserably failed. Some of those failures cost me hundreds of thousands of dollars and led to strained relationships. However, the things I learned through the process were invaluable in developing the Custom Dental model that succeeds today.

As you make changes in your business model, prepare for the fact that it will always take more effort and resources than you originally anticipated. The key is to commit to the task until it is complete. Often times you won't know until the end whether you will succeed or fail. If it is a success, enjoy the fruits of your labor. If it is a failure, reap the benefits of the education.

Edgar immediately attacked his debt with everything he had until it was gone. Later in life Parker used this principle to quickly leverage his practice into a business.

It is not my purpose in this book to share with you all the financial messes I had created before 1987, but I will say that I was very popular with dozens of creditors. Most knew my number by heart. After realizing the severity of my situation, I used a snowball technique to eliminate all of my consumer debt and much of my business debt. As I mentioned before, I have launched from the ground 11 offices. Many of our projects demand more than a $1M to open the doors. Because I took responsibility back then, I am able to borrow whatever it takes to expand Custom Dental today.

In today's climate it is easy to borrow money if you have a good track record. They may not know you as George and Jennie Parker's kids. But if they know you have always made good on your debt, the ability to leverage your business and wealth is readily available.

George Parker saw Edgar and Bessie as "silly kids" who would eventually screw up. He even discouraged them by describing their business venture as foolishness.

In 2001, I went to seven banks trying to explain my unique dental expansion model. Most of them rolled their eyes and said, *"I've never seen anything like this. Why do you think it will work? You better stick with what you know, fixing teeth."*

It is said that success is the best revenge. Today, many of those same banks are begging for my next projects. The saying is right.

Discouragement and criticism come with the accomplishment territory. You can use it as a reason to surrender or a reason to prove they are wrong. Successful folks choose option two.

Chapter Eight

LESSON LEARNED FROM CAPTAIN GRUNMARKE

Just as the wave cannot exist for itself, but is ever a part of the heaving surface of the ocean, so must I never live my life for itself, but always in the experience which is going on around me.

ALBERT SCHWEITZER

JUST before school was ending in 1884, Captain Grunmarke asked Edgar if he would like to come with him on a cod-fishing trip to the famous Grand Banks. Although he was still young and inexperienced, Edgar excitedly accepted the invitation. He had been brought up with fishermen, sailors and shipbuilders, so the way of the sea was not foreign to him.

Besides the Captain, there was a crew of three experienced fishermen. Edgar was simply listed in the ship log as "boy."

The captain's schooner was about 45 feet long. She had two masts—foremast and mainmast. There was a triangular sail at the bow called a jib. In addition, a "flying jib" and two staysails atop the foresail and mainsail could be thrown. The schooner made a pretty picture with all her sails set as she scudded across the choppy waters on the Bay of Fundy.

They set sail for the world-famous Grand Banks off Newfoundland to fish for cod and haddock. These were big, fine-tasting fish, sometimes running up to 3 feet and weighing 20 pounds.

Before they could fish for the big ones, they had to catch little ones for bait—herring and Mackerel, silvery fish 6 to 14 inches long.

The Captain explained to Edgar that he knew exactly where to fish for this bait. "You study the currents in the water and follow them. The herring feed on a microscopic sea animal and vegetation life called plankton, which drifts in the currents."

The Captain continued, as he gazed off into the sea while stroking his bewhiskered chin, *"The animal type of plankton is brought north by the Gulf Stream, and the vegetation plankton is brought south in the spring by the Arctic and Labrador currents. The currents meet and mingle off the Banks."*

Edgar was spellbound as the story teller continued. *"The plankton can't swim. They just float in the strong currents produced by the coldest water on Earth coming down from the North Pole and the warmest water on the earth coming up from the Gulf of Mexico, close to the Equator."*

The Captain added, *"The herring would swim against the current with their mouths open swallowing the plankton. And behind them would be cod, haddock and other big fish also with their mouths open ready to swallow plankton, herring and mackerel."*

Edgar thought about the plankton the rest of the day as he sat in the warm sun on the gently undulating deck of the schooner.

PRINCIPLE 9

To get anything valuable you must swim against the current.

The Captain's explanation of fish was very much like life itself. Human beings, like the fish, were swimming against the current in the ocean called life. The littlest people had their mouths open swallowing up anything smaller than themselves, and the bigger people were also swimming in the same current with their mouths wide opened, always ready to swallow, in turn, everyone else. Edgar decided that day he was going to be a big fish. Edgar enjoyed that summer immensely and learned three more important principles.

Edgar would hold tight to this principle in future years. When all his colleagues bought into the lie that advertising was unethical, Edgar swam against the current. Although swimming against that current brought him great wealth he paid the price of criticism, planned conspiracies and hundreds of thousands of dollars in legal fees.

PRINCIPLE 10

Given the choice it is better to be a big fish.

I experienced my own head-long currents the moment I changed directions with my practice in 1987. I have had classmates make comments like, *"You're not going to put one of those things in my town, are you?"* I have had to verify every testimony we used in all our advertising to the Oklahoma Dental Board because a jealous, local dentist in one of my communities filed a complaint. These are just a few examples of what happens when you swim against the current. But believe me the swim has been worth it.

You will never find success at the convenience store. In life there are really no "easy buttons." You must be willing to swim against the current to win the spoils.

Edgar would eventually implement this principle as he grew his dental empire. You will get several examples of his "Big Fish" thinking later in this book.

On our first trip to Maine, Jan and I were mesmerized by the lobster fishermen. They dragged their traps to the top of the water and grabbed the squirming creatures behind their necks and threw them into a bucket.

While watching one old weathered fisherman, we noticed that after he caught his second lobster, he had wandered over to check another trap and had forgotten to put the lid on his catch. Not wanting him to lose his prize, I casually walked up asked, *"Sir, did you realize you had forgotten to put the lid on your lobster bucket?"*

The fisherman muttered. *"I didn't forget."*

I asked, *"Aren't you afraid your catch will crawl out of the bucket while you are preoccupied with your other traps?"*

He said, *"No, son. When you have only one lobster he can climb out. So you have to put the lid on the bucket. But as soon as we add another, we don't have to worry with it anymore. If one lobster tries to escape the other one will grab him and pull him back in."*

Once I started down my growth path, I realized that I had surrounded myself with "lobsters" who were happy living in the bucket and wanted me to stay there with them. I actually had to separate

PRINCIPLE 11

There must be a place for everything and everything must be in its place.

myself from them socially and professionally and gradually seek out "Big Fish" who could mentor me.

Whether we like it or not, we determine the size of fish we are by the people we associate with and the decisions we make. It is popular today to wear a wrist band reminder with W.W.J.D. on it, which stands for "What Would Jesus Do?"

I suggest you add another band W.W.A.B.F.D., "What Would A Big Fish Do?" The next time you are faced with a decision, ask yourself the question, "What would a big fish do?" If you are not sure, there are libraries full of autobiographies of big fish. Maybe it would be smart to spend some time with them.

There was one more valuable lesson about life Edgar learned on his first deep sea-sea fishing adventure at 12 years old. Living on a boat for several months with four other men he also learned that everything should be done in a systematic way. (This principle became vital as Painless started to expand his empire.)

Structure and systems were the first things I learned in my management course in Glendale. They have become invaluable in my growth. Custom Dental has an organizational chart and an operational manual for each position in the organization. The Custom Dental structure and system is like the skeletal structure of your body. It keeps things tied together and supports all the other activities.

Systems will determine the size to which a company or practice can grow. If we do it this way one day and another the next, it is impossible to develop a team that can work together.

An eye-opening experience is to write down how you do everything in your office. If you have some fuzzy areas it is because you have no clear system to accomplish the task. Working without systems is like running a marathon in galoshes.

Chapter Nine

THE SCHOOL OF HARD KNOCKS

Success in the affairs of life often serves to hide one's abilities, whereas adversity frequently gives one an opportunity to discover them.

HORACE

THE year of 1884 marked a great crisis for the Parker family. The shipbuilding yards in Tynemouth Creek, which had been founded earlier in the century by Edgar's great-grandfather, could no longer support George Parker and his family. Sailing vessels, which the Parker family built, were being replaced by steam-driven ships and the Parker family had not made the transition.

When the shipyard failed, George attempted to open a brick-yard; however the clay deposits ran out. No more clay, no more bricks, no more brickyard business.

After the brickyard had closed, Edgar's parents decided there was little reason to stay in Tynemouth Creek. They decided to use what little money was left to move to St. Martins, a larger settlement about seven miles northeast. St. Martins was a community that Edgar had visited quite frequently while he was running his merchant business. He bought tobacco and candy at St. Martins to sell to the sailors and fishermen in Tynemouth Creek.

They left at the end of August 1884. His father hitched up the family horse and all six family members loaded into the surrey. His father, mother and baby sister, Alice, were in the front seat, and Bessie and Edgar were in the back with little Harold between them.

It was the first time in his life that Edgar had seen tears in his father's eyes. At that instant, he began to understand the impact that this event would have on the rest of his life.

In the fall of 1884, Edgar started high school at St. Martins. He was 12 1/2 years old. The transition from the very small school with one teacher in Tynemoth Creek to a large school with several teachers, whose names he couldn't even remember, was particularly difficult for Edgar. He didn't know anyone, and didn't make friends easily.

Nevertheless, the first year at St. Martins High School passed without any great mishaps. Edgar was older and generally learned how to keep out of any serious mischief. However, deep down inside, he was unhappy. He missed his home and friends at Tynemouth Creek. He did not apply himself to his studies and, consequently, his grades that year were not good.

The next year in school was even more disappointing. Jennie Parker had been having medical problems and decided to go back to Scotland, where she would stay with relatives and seek some medical relief. Jennie had been Edgar's main educational encourager. Consequently without her in the home, Edgar became more depressed and his study habits continued to deteriorate. Edgar's dad wrote to Jennie describing Edgar's despondency and continued poor scholastic performance. In reply, she suggested that under the circumstances, it would be better to send Edgar to a boarding school. The one she favored was the University of Acadia College.

The University of Acadia College was located in Wolfville, Nova Scotia, almost due east across the Bay of Fundy from Tynemouth Creek.

Edgar's father and mother both agreed this would be a great school for Edgar. They had mutually agreed that Edgar should become a Baptist minister and Acadia College was renowned for, among other things, its excellent theology school. They also thought it would be a great finishing school for Edgar because he would have the opportunity to meet the children of well-to-do families from the provinces of New Brunswick, Nova Scotia, Quebec, Newfoundland and Prince Edward Island.

When Edgar's father was completing the application for the University of Acadia College, he discovered there was an admission test, with an age minimum of 15. Edgar was 14 and had not completed some of the courses that would be covered on the test.

Edgar's father explained to him that most likely he would be enrolled in the Horton Collegiate Academy, an affiliated boarding school in Wolfville to complete the courses necessary to prepare him for Acadia College acceptance; however, he should go ahead and try for admission by sitting for the test anyway.

Edgar was not sold on this whole boarding school proposal but when his father challenged him with, *"Let's be honest, you're afraid. You haven't got the nerve to go to a school across the Bay of Fundy. You are a coward."*

"That settles it!" Edgar protested. *"I am not afraid, and I am not a coward, sir! How do I get to this school?"*

"Aren't you afraid to travel there all alone?" his father taunted. *"Don't you want me to go along with you and hold your hand so you won't get lost?"* Then realizing he was being a little too hard on the boy, George changed his manner and responded more cordially, *"You will have to take a train up to Hampton. There you will change cars for St. John and take a boat across the Bay to Digby. When you get there, you will have to take a steamer and another train to Wolfville. Do you think you could do all of that by yourself?"*

To his father's surprise, Edgar responded, *"All right, we'll see."*

On August 29, Edgar was packed up and off to Acadia College.

Although it was an arduous two-day trip to Wolfville, Edgar finally arrived at Acadia College and experienced organized education for the first time.

With only 10 pupils at the Tynemouth Creek school, there were no classes as such. At St. Martins, classes were larger, but pupils received individual attention and progressed in their studies just as rapidly, or as slowly, as the teachers found they could absorb the lessons. At Acadia College, there seemed to be hundreds of students of all ages enrolled at the University (the Horton Collegiate Academy and the Acadia Ladies' Seminary). Education was conducted on a mass-production basis.

Edgar took the entrance examination, and was assigned to the Middle Year at Horton Collegiate Academy. He found that most of the subject material he was now being taught he had already learned in New Brunswick. However, in arithmetic he had to exert himself a little. In short, there wasn't much of a challenge in his new academic environment.

There was plenty of time for sports. But the play, like the studies, was closely supervised and tightly structured. Everyone had to participate at the same time, at the same sport, starting and stopping at the same stroke of a bell. Such activity wasn't that much fun for Edgar. He was used to planning his own play—thinking up something to do, then doing it. As a result, he developed a great dislike for the excessive regimentation at Horton Collegiate. His defiance of this rigid system and his objection to the encroachment on his freedom caused him to be labeled as "rebellious and mischievous" by the sedate Horton Collegiate staff. His reputation for troublemaking landed him into more scrapes than any other student. Subsequently, this reflected in Edgar's poor Record of Deportment.

Only one of the grownups at Horton Collegiate Academy seemed to view Edgar as something more than one small cog in a great big wheel. She was Mrs. Bishop, the matron of the Horton Collegiate Academy residence where Edgar lived. She was like a mother to Edgar and the other boys in the residence and was there if any student needed to talk to someone.

Sometimes Mrs. Bishop would join the boys in the common assembly room and tell them stories as they all gathered around the large fireplace. Edgar's favorite stories were about the Acadians, the Indians who were forced to leave their home in eastern Canada. Edgar could relate to their heart-felt sorrow.

Just before his 15th birthday in March, as the warm sun returned and the snow began to melt, Edgar had reached the breaking point. He had become so unhappy that he could no longer stand life at the Horton Academy boarding school. Reciting lessons he had learned years earlier grew tiresome and boring. Playing preordained games to the tap of a bell was silly and stupid. He actually longed for the days at Tynemouth Creek when he had to get up at the crack of dawn and do an hour's worth of chores before eating breakfast.

Edgar had been taught by his parents to never waste time so

he decided to do something about his predicament. He decided he would take a direct approach and solve this problem.

He went to Mrs. Bishop and told her that he had been assigned for the upcoming winter term to the Middle Class again and nearly every subject they were giving him was "old stuff." He asked Mrs. Bishop to help him get into a class where he could really learn something new.

What Mrs. Bishop told him that day about organized education would stick with Edgar the rest of his life and influence many of the decisions and actions that molded his future.

"Edgar, you are not the first boy or girl who has rebelled at being molded into a pattern of life. This molding is necessary so that all of us will come out just like so many peas in a pod.

What you are asking—to be set ahead in your classes—is simply impossible at Acadia. When you grow up and become a man, you will find that if you try to get ahead too fast it will be equally as impossible."

Think of the Acadians, they rebelled at the edict of the King of France, who gave their land to the King of England. They fought and resisted the British authorities who came in. And what happened? They were deported and made outcasts upon the face of the earth.

You must learn to control that dynamic drive within you. You must conform. You mustn't ever try to do different than the authorities above you will allow. For if you do, then you, too Edgar, will become an outcast like the Acadians."

Edgar thought over what Mrs. Bishop said. He felt this was very unfair.

At last, he made up his mind. Come what may, outcast or not, he was not going to be made into a "pea in a pod." He resolved to be himself and exercise his own individuality! He decided that he would become a rebel and, "by hook or by crook," escape from Acadia College and Wolfville.

Edgar had learned from the fishermen at Tynemouth Creek that there were two ways to catch a fish: take them by sheer strength, by spear or by net; or capture them, using guile or one's wit as with bait or traps. He felt as though he were in a trap himself. Unlike a fish caught in a trap that cannot think, he decided to use his intellect to escape the Acadia trap.

"They wouldn't want to keep me at Acadia if they thought I was raving mad," he reasoned. *"I will just have to convince everyone that I am crazy."*

The very next morning he decided to give it a try. During the first class, he suddenly jumped up from his seat and began running around the room in circles. To make himself froth at the mouth, he slipped a small piece of caustic lye laundry soap into his mouth between his cheek and his gums. The soap tasted terrible and began to burn but he was desperate and endured it.

He kicked over chairs and hopped directly across the teacher's desk. He spun around and around, and howled like a wounded animal in pain. The frothing lye soap burned inside his mouth and gave his enactment of a raving mad person even more realism.

Edgar continued to kick, bite and scream with pain, still frothing soap bubbles from his mouth. Finally, the students in the classroom got ropes and tied him up.

As they dragged him across the floor, Edgar was able to spit out the remaining piece of soap, then he tried unsuccessfully to wipe the irritating bubbles from his lips. The students carried the squirming, moaning, sorry-looking bundle to the school infirmary, where the doctor examined him.

The doctor had him untied him and put in a chair. Edgar slumped down and let his tongue hang out one corner of his mouth, all the while panting deeply. He stared wide-eyed around the room, rolling his eyes up and down. Although the soap was gone, his mouth still hurt.

The doctor cuffed Edgar on both sides of his head, looked into his wandering eyes and said, *"Speak to me."*

Edgar began to recite the alphabet, backwards: *"ZYX-WVUTSRQPONMLkihgfe......"* as he let his voice trail off.

The doctor was a very busy man and had little patience with Edgar's behavior. He didn't want to bother with him.

After considering the perplexing situation the doctor said, *"We*

PRINCIPLE 12

If you buck the system, you risk the chance of becoming an outcast.

have no facilities here for mental cases. Send this boy home to his parents."

Relief must have shown in Edgar's eyes because the doctor became suspicious. He went over to the medicine chest, poured out an enormous amount of castor oil, held Edgar's nose and made him swallow it.

One of the teachers, Miss Stewart, was leaving on the morning train for Annapolis Royal, located about 10 kilometers west of Wolfville. There she planned to catch the night ferry to St. John, New Brunswick. She volunteered to take Edgar as far as St. John. Once there, she would get in touch with Edgar's father at St. Martins.

Even though his stomach was aching from all the castor oil and his mouth was still burning from the soap, Edgar tried to maintain his madness throughout the long journey.

After Edgar and his chaperone were on board the ferry to St. John and it had left the dock, Miss Stewart said, *"Edgar, you don't*

PRINCIPLE 13

There is always a way to change your circumstances if you are willing to do whatever it takes.

have to act crazy anymore. You are safely away from Acadia now. Have a good time on the boat. I'll not tell your father on you."

She never did. She even gave a note to his father simply saying that Edgar had been sent home because of illness. However, Edgar did not enjoy the ferry or the train ride

home, as he was still suffering from the effects of the lye soap and the physician's remedy.

Miss Stewart's note to Edgar's father seemed validated when he arrived in St. Martins. The castor oil had performed its function well. Edgar definitely looked and felt ill.

The next day was Saturday. Edgar went to Tynemouth Creek to hunt up his favorite teacher, Miss Bradshaw. He found her at home and confided in her about what actually happened at Acadia. Miss Bradshaw advised Edgar to come clean with his father. She warned him that if he didn't, he would have to live with the burden of deceit on his conscience for the rest of his life.

After considering what might happen if he followed her advice, he reckoned that he could learn to live with that deceit.

Edgar's educational experience may not have taught him much about reading, writing or arithmetic, but he did learn some other very important principles.

Mrs. Bishop warned Edgar what would happen if he tried to question or change the system. He could face condemnation and maybe even worse, such as becoming a renegade outsider. Confronted with the choice of becoming a "pea in a pod" like everyone else, or risk being an outcast, Edgar chose the latter. That choice enabled him to be one of the most successful dentists in history, at the price of also being misunderstood, and often labeled as a dental outcast.

I have already mentioned that I am not well received in most dental circles. I don't know if it is fear or confusion that repels people from me, but I have learned to live with the truth that they are the ones with the problem. I'm just fine.

If you think your successful journey will be somehow void of this consequence, you probably still believe in the tooth fairy. Many potential greats have fallen to the wayside because the skin they wore was too thin.

Edgar was trapped at the Acadia College; forced to pursue a career he had no interest in, Baptist minister; taking classes he felt were a waste of time; and being controlled by a silly system of conformity and bells. How many other children in that school felt the same way? How many were actually willing to do something about it? How many would risk acting a fool, swallowing lye soap and taking castor oil to escape?

Edgar was a boy and a man of action, which eventually contributed to his illustrious future.

In 2001, I was attempting to launch my first model expansion. There was only one workable piece of property for sale in the targeted community. Its main problem was that it had no access to sewer service.

I checked around town. The closest sewer access was 600 feet away, which meant I would have to get an easement between two adjacent property owners. If overcoming the added expense of laying a 600-foot of sewer line was a speed bump, getting an easement from the adjacent neighbors was like climbing to the top of Pike's Peak.

After many dead ends I finally made an appointment with Charles Malzahn, the owner of the largest employer in the community, Ditch Witch. Charles employed about 800 of the 5,000 residents in Perry, Oklahoma, and he was very active in the community.

When I was escorted into his office, I met a rather small-framed, down-home gentleman who appeared to be about 70. After a few kind formalities, I pled my case and asked if he knew anyone who could help.

I said, *"Mr. Malzahn, I am a dentist and I want to improve your community by building a beautiful dental building on the main thoroughfare into your community. I want to provide World Class Dental Experiences for your employees and their families. However, I have run into what seems to be an insurmountable challenge. I need your help."* I went on to explain my challenge.

When I finished he said, *"Well, Doctor Brown, it sounds like you need a little help from the city planner and the city council."*

He picked up the phone, made a call to one of his managers and within a few moments I was shaking the hand of a city council member.

Three city council meetings and two months later the sewer easement was approved. The rest is history. Had I let this obstacle block our first expansion attempt, there may not have been a Custom Dental that has successfully partnered with 11 dentists and employs 80 support staff in two states.

At your next dental meeting or social event, listen to the common conversation. *"My dental assistant is a klutz." "I think my office manager is stealing from me." "That insurance company is going to send me to bankruptcy court."*

What you will hear are problems with no solutions. And when you try to offer one, they want to hold tight to the problem, like the

Charley Brown, blanket-toting character, Linus. You'll hear responses like, *"That may work for you, but my practice is different."*

It reminds me of the story about the ole boy back home who went to see his friend. When he arrived, he found his friend peacefully rocking in his favorite chair on the covered front porch. Next to him was his favorite companion, Duke, a 10-year-old blood hound.

After a few pleasantries, their conversation was interrupted with a blood curdling howl that only a bloodhound can make. The visitor was shocked and asked *"What's wrong with Duke?"*

His friend casually answered, *"Oh, Duke? He's just lying on a nail."*

His guest was shocked at his casualness and asked, *"Why doesn't he move?"*

The friend said, *"I don't think it hurts enough to move and I think he just likes to howl about it."*

The world is filled with Dukes who seem to enjoy the suffering of lying on their nail, as well as the sound of their own howling. Those who succeed in dentistry, or in life, spend little time complaining about the problems they face along the way. Instead, they spend their time searching for a way to escape their trap.

Chapter Ten

PARKER GETS HIS FIRST REAL JOB, A LIFE- CHANGING EXPERIENCE

"Expect the best. Prepare for the worst. Capitalize on what comes."

ZIG ZIGLAR

IN March 1887, just before his 15th birthday, Edgar returned to St. Martins and his family. He was pleased to see everyone because he hadn't been back since leaving in August of 1886. And, in fact, hadn't seen his mother since September of 1885. When the topic of the Acadia experience came up, Edgar sheepishly tried to change the subject.

Even after his initial failure at Acadia College and his father's attempt at securing him a position in a local mercantile business, Edgar's parents still hoped that he would come to his senses and become a Baptist minister. Since the Baptist church in St. Martins had a seminary, the Parker's decided to give their son one last shot at becoming "a man of the cloth."

Edgar entered the seminary in the fall of 1887. By the spring of 1888, he was once again rejected from an educational institution for bucking the system and playing pranks. Now what would happen?

He did not dare go home and face his parents. He couldn't tell them he had been expelled from seminary. Their hopes for him to become a Baptist preacher had vanished. It appeared to him that he had only one choice: get as far away from St. Martins as he could, as soon as he could.

Edgar talked over this unpleasant situation with one of his seminary accomplices. It was decided he would approach a gentleman in Moncton, a community 139 kilometers northeast of St. Martins. It was hoped this man might have some work for him. The accomplice gave Edgar a note to the man and even lent him some money to buy a train ticket.

It was late April when Edgar arrived in Moncton. He lost no time hunting down the man who could provide a job. He wanted to start making money as soon as possible so he could pay back his friend. He had already experienced being in debt and didn't like it at all.

The job turned out to be peddling notions such as tobacco, coffee, calico, needles, pins, sugar and housewares, from farm to farm. His employer was John MacKenzie, a shrewd and honest Scots trader who sold goods to salesmen travelling throughout the countryside.

The note his friend had hastily scribbled told Mr. MacKenzie that Edgar belonged to the famous shipbuilding-and-sea- captain Parker family and that he was worthy of hire. Mr. MacKenzie decided that the "Parker" name was good enough for him to chance. To test the young man's honesty and trading ability, he offered to start Edgar out with a horse, a wagon and a stock of merchandise.

He told Edgar that, while peddling wasn't a fancy occupation, it was an honest way to make a living, as it filled a genuine need for people who lived in remote areas with no railroads and very few stores. Edgar was to receive 10% of everything he sold, plus his expenses. Out of this profit, he could pay for the old horse, rickety wagon and merchandise.

Edgar was quite nervous as he drove up to the first farmhouse to offer his wares. He almost hoped that the residents would not be home. However, he quickly found that he was indeed welcome. What he didn't realize at first was that he not only provided needed products, but he was also a source of news for these isolated farmers. None of the country people he called on would allow him to pay for a meal nor would they accept his money for a place to sleep at night. He was treated more like a guest than a country peddler.

Not many of his customers had actual cash, but they did have plenty of things to trade or barter. Chickens, eggs, live pigs, sacks of grain, hams and sides of bacon, preserves, jam and all sorts of home-grown fruits and vegetables were swapped for the manufactured products that Edgar brought to them. When Edgar reached a lum-

PRINCIPLE 14
Those who succeed always find the silver lining in every cloud.

bering camp, he could quickly turn those items into cash or he would sell them directly to the stores or shops located in a nearby town near the railroad.

He also discovered that, although he made a living out of peddling, he couldn't expect to make more than that because of the time he wasted traveling from place to place.

Almanacs were the most popular item he carried. They were the favorite reading material for everyone. The almanac contained chapters on astrology; it had horoscopes; it forecasted the weather for a year and told farmers what time of the moon to plant and harvest their crops. It gave recipes for cooking and concocting medicines for all types of ailments. It was full of quotations, homespun philosophy, wise sayings and jokes. So when Edgar sold entirely out of coffee, tea, tobacco, women's sewing supplies, bolts of calico and gingham, crockery, toys, almanacs and whatever else he might have, he drove

PRINCIPLE 15
Successful business owners learn to do more in less time.

his horse and wagon to the nearest railroad town, sent his earnings to Mr. MacKenzie and asked him to send back an especially large order of almanacs with his next order.

It took Edgar a week to dispose of the items that he had taken as barter from the farmers and lumbermen. At the same time, he did a little trading of his own. He swapped his "crow bait," giving sacks of grain and cured hams "to boot," for a fine, glossy-coated black stallion.

When the train finally arrived with a large packing case addressed to "Edgar R. Parker," he was surprised to discover that there was nothing in it except almanacs, 500 of them. He assumed the other goods he ordered had gone astray. There was no telling when they might show up. He felt dejected, realizing he couldn't make a living selling one almanac at a time to farmers. And to make matters worse he had sent all his earnings to Mr. MacKenzie to apply as a payment for the horse and wagon. What should he do?

Feeling very downcast, Edgar looked through one of the almanacs. They were an extra-fine edition with a cloth cover. He wasn't sure what to charge for them but he thought they were surely worth one dollar.

As he was pondering his circumstances, a train coming from lumber country pulled into the station. Out of the train poured a crowd of lumberjacks who had just completed their spring work in the woods. He knew they would have money just begging to be spent.

PRINCIPLE 16

If you want your message heard you need to start it with a headline.

Zig Ziglar, the famous motivational speaker, most accurately captured Edgar's emotions at that moment when he made reference to his cookware salesman days. *"Those folks had my money in their pockets and it was my job to make sure they got their cookware in exchange."*

Edgar jumped on top of the packing case containing the almanacs and shouted, *"Gentlemen, please listen to me. Step over here, please, and let me show you something of greatest interest."*

The men approached, hoping for some fun, laughing and carrying on, while being very curious to see what the young boy had.

"I have 500 almanacs here," he said.

All eyes turned on him. A hush fell over the noisy crowd. Edgar drew in his breath and said, in a much louder and clearer voice that was gaining confidence. *"You all know what almanacs are. Sure you do. But you have never seen an almanac like this before. Two hundred pages full of excitement. And a clothe cover to boot, yes Siree! I am practically giving them away for only a dollar per copy."*

PRINCIPLE 17

If you want to influence a crowd, influence the influencer.

A tall, young Scandinavian seemed to be the leader of the group. He stood head-high above the rest. Edgar had heard one of the others call him "Chris." He singled him out, looked him straight in the eye and called out, *"You, Chris! You take one of these almanacs and just look at it."*

He grinned, took one and said, *"What does a lumberjack want with an almanac?"* Laughter abounded among the group.

"It tells you how to write love letters," Edgar winked and replied with a chuckle. *"And it's got a lot of astrology in it. It will tell you what kind of girl you ought to marry."*

"I already got a wife," said Chris.

The crowd again roared with laughter.

"Then get an almanac for her," Edgar quickly retorted. *"This is the biggest and best almanac ever published. Send it to your wife! She'll love you for your thoughtfulness. She will be proud to have the finest and biggest almanac in town! Nobody else, not even the richest people, will have a grander almanac. She will look forward to seeing you soon."*

PRINCIPLE 18

Sell the benefits, not the features.

Chris climbed up on the wagon beside Edgar. He turned to the crowd while laughing.

"The kid's all right," he yelled out. *"You fellers who've got wives, you better buy an almanac. Those of you who have sweethearts ought to buy one, too. And, if you haven't got a sweetheart, then you better learn how to write love letters!*

I like this kid! He's got the gift of gab. And he knows good horseflesh; look at that fine stallion! I am paying a dollar for this almanac.

Everybody buy an almanac, or else!" He ordered them, adding, *"Or else you will have to lick me."*

Everybody bought one. No one wanted to take on Chris.

Clutching their almanacs in their big, dirty hands, the lumberjacks milled away up town to spend their remaining wages. Meanwhile, Edgar counted the money he had collected in his hat and found he had taken in $29, all within only a half hour!

Edgar was beginning to realize that he could sell and he had a special knack for communicating his message to a group.

There is more to this almanac story but there are so many principles to be learned at this point I must take a break to point them out to you.

When Edgar received the shipment of 500 almanacs, he only momentarily considered his misfortune. He immediately changed his business model to adapt to the circumstances, when he decided to use the "one-to-many sales approach" instead of his previous "one-to-one" method.

How many times are we faced with a challenge and either retreat or try to overcome it using old methods? There is a saying, "Necessity is the mother of invention."

It always amazes me when I find a dentist who works from nine to four and can't seem to get busy. Or he can't get a new patient in for two weeks yet his practice is in the bottom 20%. They say insanity is doing the same thing over and over, while expecting different results.

PRINCIPLE 19

When you make them laugh it lubricates their wallet.

When I supercharged my practice, one of the things I did was to adjust my schedule. We started taking appointments at 7 A.M. and staying until 7 P.M. a few nights a week.

In Edgar's case, he figured out he could not make a living selling almanacs one at a time so he employed group selling.

I am always shocked at dentists who complain about not making enough money, yet they are convinced they cannot increase their speed or efficiency. They use their slowness as some kind of justification for thoroughness. In most cases, many of the things they are doing to slow them down are not improving the quality of the care for the patient. Most people would say *"If you can do my root canal in 1 to 2 hours or 10 to 20 minutes, I'll take the latter."* There are several automated endo classes being offered across the country. There is no excuse for not increasing your speed and efficiency in every service you offer. When you do that, everyone wins.

Another point about this principle is that when Edgar was faced with his problem, he stepped up and presented his case to a crowd.

Why do we feel it is the patient's obligation to find us hiding in our little offices? There are numerous opportunities to speak to groups either at their meetings or by holding an event at your own office. I know public speaking is a hurdle for some. It was for me. But when I decided to grow my practice I realized I would have to do things that were uncomfortable. Comfortable was keeping me broke.

I read everything I could get my hands on about public speaking, watched the experts deliver, jumped up on my own box and stumbled forward. And like Edgar, I eventually learned how to influence others from the front of the room. Let me tell you how he did that.

There were two parts to Edgar's headline. He identified his target by addressing them as "gentlemen." If he had started jabbering about the almanacs without addressing them directly, they may have ignored him and meandered on in to town.

Next he captured their attention by creating curiosity. He suggested he had something that they would be interested in seeing.

I think much can be learned from Edgar's example and applied in your treatment plan presentation. Having partnered with, mentored, employed and trained hundreds of dentists, I have noticed that most dentists are weak at communicating necessary care to patients. They never totally connect. The consumer doesn't seem to understand what they need and why it is important to address their issues. The outcome is frustrating for both.

At Custom Dental, we have an 11-step, choreographed script that covers these communication principles.

But what if you just address the patient by their name? What if you relate to who they are? What if you build curiosity before you deliver the plan? What could happen if you relate these ideas to your case presentation?

"Mary, you being a busy mom, I am sure you are going to be interested in what I found during your examination today."

Edgar noticed who seemed to be the leader of the group, called him out and did his best to sell him on the almanac. Then he let Chris sell the group.

Have you ever gone to a dental meeting and picked up a great idea you wanted to implement but then the idea died quickly when you tried to get your team behind it? You didn't use this principle.

I used it to build and steer my dental team as I transformed my practice. I still use it today with our Custom Dental Support Team. Any time I want to initiate a new concept in our company, I always have a meeting with my influencers first. Once I am good with them, we go to the group with the idea. When I present my proposal to the group they all observe the body language of the influencer. As soon as they get a positive read from them, they buy into the new concept. Sometimes I even have the influencer present the idea.

Can you identify your influencers? Can you influence your influencers? *How to Win Friends and Influence People* and *Influence: The Psychology of Persuasion* are two of my favorite books on this subject.

If you noticed, Edgar seldom mentioned the almanac without sharing how it would influence its owner's outcome. Another twist to this principle is that Edgar took a stab at the purpose for which he thought the lumberjacks would use the almanac, and then he adjusted his delivery to show them how owning an almanac could help them achieve it. It could help them find love or make their lovers proud of them.

Trying to sell dental care without knowing what is important to the patient (selling the features, not the benefits) and attempting

PRINCIPLE 20

If you think everyone will be excited about your success, you are wrong.

to influence the patient with logic is a formula for failure. Believe me, I tried it for years. No matter how long you talk about the quality of the denture material, it won't make near the impact as mentioning how the odor-resistant material will give them confidence in a crowd.

When I discovered this principle, the world became my oyster.

"Mary, I understand you are a busy mom with four kids. I know everyone depends on you to get them to games, school and other activities. You don't have time to be down. That is why I wanted to mention what I found in your exam and why we need to address these issues. Or you could face some very time- consuming consequences soon."

Okay, so let's get back to Edgar and his hat full of money and see what else we can learn from his first real job experience.

(Back to Edgar selling almanacs.)

Arriving on the next day's train was another large box containing Edgar's regular peddling goods. He also found a letter at the post office from Mr. MacKenzie. It explained that the expensive looking almanacs he had sent were a lot he picked up quite cheaply. He would be charging Edgar 5 cents a copy and he thought they could be sold for a quarter each. What a windfall!!

The following day, Edgar headed for a county fair in a nearby town. He parked his rig on a crowded street, jumped up on his wagon and commenced his sales pitch. He spoke about the almanacs and about the other wonderful items he had for sale. People gathered in groups to listen. Edgar found that the best way to hold the crowd's attention was to read selected jokes and limericks out of the almanac. If he could get them laughing, they would be more apt to spend their money.

Edgar eventually perfected a good sales pitch that he delivered from the back of his wagon whenever he could amass a crowd. By the end of three months, he had made enough money to pay Mr. MacKenzie in full for the old horse, the rickety wagon and the stock of goods.

Edgar discovered happy people are better customers.

I found out that happy patients accept more care. As I mentioned before, I was 24 when I saw my first private practice patient. I was very self conscious about my youth and tried hard to overcome it with a serious demeanor. I even grew a beard.

After discovering this principle, I consciously started smiling. Eventually, I learned a few appropriate humorous comments and used them in predictably tense moments.

When Mary would ask, *"Well, how much is all of this going to cost, doc?"*

I would say *"Well Mary, that's a great question and Rene will be in here soon to answer it. But don't worry, I don't think you will need to knock off a Quick Stop to pay for it. If you do, don't worry, I'll drive the getaway car."* Then I'd finish with a BIG SMILE.

(Back to Edgar.)

Edgar was so proud to have his own business. In only three short months he was out of debt with money in his pocket. He couldn't stand it. Edgar decided to drive his rig down to St. John to show off his outfit to his parents. He just knew his recent success would finally make them proud.

The peddler's outfit that Edgar wore when driving up to the front of his parent's house was as showy as money could buy. He had outfitted his spirited, black stallion with a silver-mounted harness, set with two black ostrich plumes waving from a special collar. His wagon had been painted bright red with yellow striping; and on both sides of the wagon his name, **"Edgar R. Parker,"** was displayed in big gold lettering. He wore a pearl-gray hat with a tall crown and a wide brim, a fancy green sequenced vest and an even fancier bright red silk tie. He had let his black hair grow long and sported a black Vandyke beard.

Imagine the surprise of Edgar's parents at, and their reaction to this gaudily dressed horse peddler. He was a far cry from the son they had sent to St. Martins to prepare to become a Baptist minister.

Edgar's mother was so glad to see him that she hugged and repeatedly kissed him and pretended not to notice his garish appearance. His father was dumfounded and said nothing, but simply gawked in astonishment. Then, to regain in his senses, he rushed out the door, quickly jumped into Edgar's wagon and hastily drove it around the house into the barn. Edgar could hear him muttering under his breath as he slammed the barn door.

His mother lead Edgar to the parlor where she shared with him what they had done when they found out that he had left the seminary in St. Martins. They weren't sure what had become of him after he went to Moncton. They had advertised in the newspaper all over the province asking Edgar to come back and letting him know all was forgiven.

His father came into the parlor, quite vexed, but Edgar was oblivious to his father's agitation as he happily and excitedly told his parents about his peddling activities, about how he had made enough money to pay for the wagon, a horse and a full load of merchandise. He proudly announced that he had no debts and he had money in his pockets. He was bursting with pride. But that was short lived.

His father couldn't contain himself any longer. He literally shook all over, and his face turned red. He looked as if he were going to burst. Edgar realized that he had never seen his father so upset.

"You ought to be horsewhipped" he yelled, shaking with rage.

"Now George," Jennie pleaded quietly, *"you advertised and promised to forgive him."*

"All right!" said his father, calming down a bit, *"But there will be no more disgrace to the Parker name with that red painted wagon going around New Brunswick with our son dressed up like a nincompoop, looking like a circus freak at a side show. Peddling! A Parker peddler! I will not have it!"*

"He's only 16!" defended his mother.

"It makes no difference." His father snorted back.

"He is going to get out of those outlandish clothes, shave that beard, get his hair cut and go back to school to become a minister. I'm going to paint out the Parker name on that wagon and sell it."

"There's no disgrace in peddling!" Edgar angrily shouted back at his father. *"It's an honest way to earn a living, and that's all I care about. I may only be 16, but I've had three summers at sea, and I'm rated an able seaman! You are not going to force me to become a minister! I'll run away first! I am going to live my own life."*

Fortunately, his mother quickly stepped in and quieted them down before they came to blows.

The next day, his father carried out his threat. He took Edgar's wagon downtown and had it auctioned, together with his most treasured horse, the silver-mounted harness and his entire stock of merchandise.

That night, seething with injustice, Edgar carried out his own threat. He left home, after writing his mother a note, sadly telling her he would be all right and not to worry because he was running away to the sea. Little did anyone know that this new chapter in Edgar's life would open the door to him becoming a dentist.

Edgar was so convinced that his success would impress his parents and make them happy, he drove days to tell them.

In 2001, when I presented my idea to bankers, they looked at me like I had spinach in my teeth. I made my presentation to six before I found one who would loan me money.

Today when I go back to my dental class reunions or other dental meetings, I usually find myself trying to explain what I do. Most eyes glaze over, with no comment forthcoming.

It has been said there are three kinds of folks: those who make it happen, those who watch it happen and those who wonder what happened. Your road to success will be lined with those who will question, jeer and criticize your efforts. Don't let them distract you. "The dogs will bark, but the caravan must move on."

Chapter Eleven

WHAT DOESN'T KILL YOU
MAKES YOU STRONGER

"The best executive is the one who has sense enough to pick good men to do what he wants done, and self-restraint enough to keep from meddling with them while they do it."

THEODORE ROOSEVELT

WITH money left in his pocket, Edgar bought a train ticket to Quebec. Upon arrival, he immediately signed on as an extra deck hand on one of his uncle's vessels, the *Nellie Parker*, which was leaving the next day with a full cargo for Bridgetown, Barbados. She would unload, take on another cargo and be back within a month. Although he had made many coastline excursions, this would be Edgar's first chance on the open sea.

One day after returning from Barbados and while wandering through the wharves, Edgar spied the most magnificent sailing ship he had ever seen, the *Cyprus*. He had heard about her because his uncle, Raymond Parker, had been her first captain. On family get-togethers at Tynemouth Creek, Raymond frequently shared stories of the Cyprus and her speedy trips across the ocean. These fast passages made Uncle Raymond and the *Cyprus* the talk of seafaring men all over the North Atlantic. She was a legendary vessel.

A sailor on the wharf told him that the *Cyprus* was presently commanded by Captain William Steeves. Edgar boldly walked up the gangplank and asked if he could see Captain Steeves.

When asked why, Edgar replied, *"I am a nephew of Captain Raymond Parker, the first captain of the Cyprus."*

Captain Steeves immediately summoned Edgar to his cabin.

"Young man," he said, *"you come from a remarkable seafaring family. I know them all, your father George Parker, and his five brothers Captain Raymond Parker, Captain James Parker, Captain William Parker, Captain Thomas Parker and John Parker, the ship chandler in New York. Some family! Your father builds ships, your four sea-captain uncles sail' em and your uncle John outfits' em!"*

"Now, what about you, young sir? What are you to make of yourself?"

"I would like to ship before the mast on the **Cyprus** *under you, sir!"* blurted out Edgar.

"So! Another generation of Parkers to become sea captains. Is that your idea boy?" chuckled Captain Steeves, with a twinkle in his eye.

"Why not, sir?" replied Edgar, with self-assurance. *"My Uncle Raymond had his master's ticket before he was 21 years old. He told me so himself."*

"How old are you?" What education do you have? Have you any sailing experience?"

"I am 16, almost 17, sir," Edgar answered excitedly. *"I've had a high school education lacking 1 month. When I was 12 years old, I sailed as a fisherman on the Grand Banks with Captain Grunmarke. The last three summers, I sailed on the coasting ships the A.P. Emerson and the For and After to Maine, Boston, New York, Philadelphia and Baltimore. I also sailed for a short time to Barbados on the Nellie Parker. I am an able seaman, sir, and if you will tell me what books to get and help me with them, I can learn navigation, sir."*

PRINCIPLE 21

A successful leader knows the strengths of each individual on the team and leverages it.

"There's a lot of difference between sailing on coastal vessels and deep-sea sailing, young man," scoffed Captain Steeves. *"We're sailing deep sea, from Quebec to Argentina. Crews on coasters are tough but comparatively decent men. The kind we have to take on for deep-sea sailing are the scum of the waterfront. Many are fugitives from the law. They are so low that the coasters have kicked them out; men with weak minds but strong backs; stupid, cruel and hard men. Harder men than you would ever believe."*

Captain Steeves paused, allowing what he just said sink in.

Edgar appeared nervous.

"That's who you'll have for crewmates. Do you still want to sail deep sea before mast?"

"Yes, sir," Edgar replied somewhat apprehensively, while shifting his weight from one foot to the other.

"All right," said the Captain. *"See Mr. Saunders, the first mate."*

Edgar found Mr. Saunders and asked about signing on the *Cyprus*. When the Shipping Master came aboard later that day, Edgar became an able seaman for the cruise, which he discovered would probably take about a year.

He helped with the final loading of cargo of lumber and hardware and with the other preparations for sailing. During this time, he began to see firsthand what Captain Steeves meant when he warned Edgar about what type of crew that a captain had to hire for this type of deep-sea sailing.

Before he left Quebec, Edgar wrote a long letter to his mother, telling her what he had done, but he didn't mail it until the day they left port.

Later in his life Parker reflected that this trip would teach him many principles about life that helped him pioneer what he called "group dentistry." So let's move on and see what they were.

PRINCIPLE 22

A successful practice is framed with a set of functional systems.

Once at sea, Edgar found the crew members were all that Captain Steeves had said, and more. They were a tough, motley and rough lot of natives from many countries. They were always quarreling with each other, quick to use their teeth, knives, marlinspikes, clubs and fists.

Although he was the only boy, he had dared to call himself an able seaman. They knew that he was studying navigation to become an officer. As a result, the crew seemed to resent Edgar for having a spark of ambition, and they did all they could to make his life miserable.

The boatswain's mate piled the most unpleasant and hardest work on Edgar, to make him earn his "salt junk," the name for the barreled salted beef that was the sailor's principal food.

After leaving Quebec, their first stop was Barbados. They unloaded their cargo of lumber and hardware from Quebec and reloaded with sugar, indigo, cotton, tobacco and ginger.

From Barbados they rounded the bulge of Brazil and landed at Rio de Janerio. It was one of the finest and most beautiful harbors in the world. The official language spoken in Brazil was Portuguese.

They unloaded their cargo from Barbados in Rio de Janerio and reloaded with Brazilian brandy, coffee, medicinal herbs and rare hardwoods and headed to Buenos Aires, Argentina.

The port of Buenos Aires was not only on the seacoast but also on the River Plate. At the time Edgar was there, ships drawing more than 16 feet of water had to anchor 7 or 8 miles offshore and discharge their cargo in smaller transport boats.

Edgar was given shore leave along with the other crew members. They rowed the ship's longboat ashore to the inner channels, where the water was barely deep enough for smaller boats.

It was early December, 1888. Because Argentina is south of the equator it was late spring and the climate was like early June in the America Carolinas.

As soon as the crew landed on shore, they made a beeline for the many waterfront dives, saloons and dance halls in Buenos Aires. They all had pay in their pockets. Edgar stuck his nose in two or three of these dives just long enough to whiff their smell, but they were too rank for him. These dives were no different from the other waterfront dives that he had seen in many other ports, except maybe these were a little dirtier and the painted women only spoke Spanish.

He left the waterfront area and went up to the business district. It was much cleaner there. All the signs on the buildings were in Spanish, so he couldn't read them. He wandered about, trying to get back to the waterfront, when suddenly he found himself caught in the cross fire of one of those insurgent fights. A bullet intended for an enemy hit him and went through his right leg. This would be his first trip to the hospital.

Meanwhile, the *Cyprus* sailed away and left him in the hospital in Buenos Aires. When he was released, he signed on an old ship anchored in the harbor, the *Richard Peterson*, a Canadian registered vessel. He got a job standing watch on the ship.

During one morning watch, Edgar witnessed four men get their throats slit on the vessel anchored nearby. Edgar decided that he wanted to live, so during the night and morning watches he would hoist himself halfway up the mast, tie himself to it and try to catch sleep out of harm's way. This may not have made him a very good lookout, but it probably saved his life.

On another shore leave in Buenos Aires, he saw a native drinking some wine from a long-necked glass bottle. Edgar was very thirsty and warm, so he went over and took a swig of wine from the bottle. After having several gulps, he reached into his pocket, but couldn't find any money. He suddenly remembered he had left his money back at the ship. He tried to explain to the fellow that he would go back to the ship and return with the money to pay him, but the native didn't understand English.

Edgar turned to go back to the ship and hadn't gone 20 feet when the fellow called over to a gaucho on horseback. This man threw a lasso over Edgar's head and started his horse running. Edgar was dragged three blocks before the gaucho let him go. One side of Edgar's face and one hand had the skin peeled back.

Edgar was arrested and taken to a judge, who only spoke Spanish. He was sentenced to serve four days in jail. While there, he was told by another young sailor and a fellow prisoner that the police were in the habit of sending prisoners up-country to work. No one spoke English and the guards worked the prisoners like slaves. If a prisoner resisted orders, they were killed.

The captain from the *Richard Peterson* finally found Edgar in prison and had him released. From there, they sailed to Barbados.

After the *Richard Peterson* returned to Buenos Aires, Edgar, having nothing to do, was walking along the top of the ship's rail when he lost his balance and fell overboard into the contaminated harbor, nearly drowning. Before being rescued, he swallowed a large amount of brackish harbor water. Edgar became very sick with dengue fever. His fever was so severe, and Edgar was so ill, that the captain had him admitted back into the local hospital. It was during this rather lengthy stay in the hospital that Edgar observed, for the first time, how the physicians strutted around importantly in their white coats. They ordered everyone about frequently and dosed their patients with castor oil. It seemed in this environment, their word was law.

While Edgar was convalescing there, the *Cyprus* returned to Buenos Aires and Captain Steeves found him. Once Edgar was dismissed from the hospital, Captain Steeves gave him back his previous job.

Edgar had learned it was much safer to stay on board, so he didn't spend much time ashore after that. He used most of his free time on the *Cyprus* studying navigation and the methods of loading and unloading cargo.

Captain Steeves noticed Edgar's seriousness and began to mentor him. He even allowed him to stand in when the second mate went missing.

Once Captain Steeves said to Edgar, "*A smart officer can make a faster sailing if he studies the men in his watch and discovers what each man can do best. Some men can steer better than others; put them at the wheel. Some are naturally handy with a needle; let them patch and sew the sails. Some are best aloft; use them aloft.*"

On another occasion, Captain Steeves explained to Edgar the reason for the great success of the sailing firm. "*My boy, our basic secret is organization,*" reflected the captain, "*organization ashore and afloat.*"

Things were going good for Edgar. He was earning the trust of the captain and first mate, all the while learning every detail on how to run a successful ship. However, things were about to change.

One of the sailors on the *Cyprus*, a fellow named Pete, was spreading a rumor that Edgar had gotten the second mate drunk in Buenos Aires so he would miss the ship launching and Edgar could get his position. When Edgar heard the rumor from another sailor he told the informant not to spread it any further. The informant also told Edgar that Pete was out to get him.

Edgar simply ignored the matter and quickly forgot the warning. One dark night, when Edgar was threading his way through the inspection of the gear, someone suddenly sprang out of the darkness and viciously hit him from the back on his spine with a jib-sheet pin, a four-foot long metal pole. It knocked Edgar unconscious as well as damaging his vertebrae. When he came to, he was in his cabin. He stayed in his bunk, suffering pain the entire trip from Buenos Aires to Barbados. What was worse, the lower portion of his body was paralyzed. He could not walk.

When the *Cyprus* reached Barbados, Captain Steeves had Edgar transferred to the hospital, where the doctors confirmed his vertebrae trauma but were uncertain how serious it was. Once again, Edgar took notice of the doctors walking around in their white coats and receiving a lot of respect.

The doctors put splints on Edgar's injured back and bound him tightly with bandages as they begrudgingly allowed him to return to the ship. It was leaving Barbados headed to St. John, where Edgar's parents now lived. Captain Steeves felt if he could get Edgar to St. John, his parents could take care of him.

As a result of the unceasing pain, Edgar lost 60 pounds, dropping to just barely over 100. One thing all the doctors recommended was that Edgar quit the sea. At the very best, they said, it would be many years before he would walk and regain the strength necessary for such a hard life.

PRINCIPLE 23
The principle of Have, Do, Be.

The pain in his back never ceased during the long voyage home.

There are three principles that Edgar learned during this episode of his life. I will point out two now and address the third later on in Edgar's story.

Captain Steeves was a good captain, leader and mentor. Engineering wasn't the only reason the *Cyprus* was so famously fast. Captain Steeves knew where to position his men and get the best results.

This principle reminds me of a story I once heard from John Maxwell, a famous speaker and leadership coach.

"Once upon a time, the animals decided they should do something meaningful to meet the problems of the new world. So they organized a school.

They adopted an activity curriculum of running, climbing, swimming, and flying. To make it easier to administer, all the animals took all of the subjects.

The duck was excellent at swimming, in fact, he was better than his instructor was! However, he made only passing grades in flying, and was very poor in running. Since he was so slow in running, he had to drop swimming and stay after school to practice running. This caused his webbed feet to be badly worn so he became only average in swimming. But 'average' was quite acceptable, therefore nobody worried about it, except the duck.

The rabbit started at the top of his class in running, but developed a nervous twitch in his leg muscles because he had so much makeup work to do in swimming.

The squirrel was excellent in climbing, but he encountered constant frustration in flying classes because his teacher made him start from the ground up instead of from the treetop down. He developed 'charley horses' from overexertion so he only got a 'C' in climbing and a 'D' in running.

The eagle was a problem child and was severely disciplined for being a non-conformist. In climbing classes, he beat all the others to the top, but insisted on using his own way to get there!"

This silly story illustrates that everybody is a "10" at something but if you put them in the wrong position in your organization you will frustrate them, wear calluses on the their feet and, at best, get an average performance.

There are several skills necessary in running a successful dental practice: eye-hand coordination, organization, sales acumen and hospitality, to list just a few. I found that when I placed the right person in their strength zone, our ship sailed much more smoothly and at a faster pace.

Captain Steeves shared with Edgar that not only placing the right folks in the right spots was important, but those right folks working in the right spots, worked inside a set of systems on and off the sea to ensure maximum efficiency.

As I have mentioned before, Custom Dental has an organizational board that assigns everyone in the office to a post. Within each post there are several responsibilities and each of those responsibilities are spelled out in step-by-step detail.

Over the years I have noticed it is not uncommon for a dentist to have a set of steps to use to complete a root canal or prepare a tooth for a crown, but the process of how a lab case is handled, tracked and returned from the lab is as inconsistent as the Oklahoma weather.

There are a thousand systems that need to be developed, trained and monitored in a dental practice to make sure it is running at maximum capacity. Most dentists don't have a clue how things get done, making them victims in their own practices.

Chapter Twelve

PARKER'S FIRST GLIMPSE
INSIDE DENTISTRY

"Seek first to understand before attempting to be understood."

STEPHEN COVEY

EDGAR'S return to St. John, Canada, in the spring of 1889 marked another turning point in his life. During Edgar's year-and-a-half absence, Jennie Parker had been to New York and had some impacted wisdom teeth surgically removed. Afterwards she developed a chronic sinus infection that persisted even after multiple trips to various specialists. On her way back to St. John she stopped off to visit a friend, Mary Baker Eddy, in Boston. Mary was a devout Christian Scientist. Jennie was desperate for a cure. It was never fully known whether it was Jennie's newly acquired religious faith or her own healing powers that miraculously healed her sinus infection soon after that visit. As for Edgar, he spent the entire summer in the hospital convalescing; suffering constant, severe pain and unable to move. In those days, the St. John hospital had no x-rays, no chiropractors, no allopaths, no homeopaths and no osteopaths. There were only medical doctors, who apparently had little knowledge of what to do to help him.

PRINCIPLE 24

Whenever you have the choice, choose affluent neighborhoods.

In desperation to treat Edgar's ailing vertebrae Dr. Holden, a physician in St. John, one day proceeded to jump on his back with a pair of sea boots. Edgar promptly passed

PRINCIPLE 25
Word of mouth has always been the most influential source of marketing.

out from the pain. Still no cure.

Since he was confined to bed rest in the hospital all summer, Edgar had time to think. He considered what would have happened if he would have completed his studies at Acadia College and had become a Baptist minister. What a boring life, stuck in some small Maritime town.

PRINCIPLE 26
Treat everyone like the lady of the house.

He fondly remembered the excitement of peddling his goods off the back of his wagon and speaking to crowds. And oh, how he missed that beautiful black stallion all decked out in his silver-studded harness!

Edgar also reflected on the lessons he had learned at sea with Captain Steeves, about how to assign people to do what they do best and how to skillfully manage with systems.

When spring had turned into summer, Edgar was sent home. Nothing further could be done for him at the hospital. Even under his

PRINCIPLE 27
Know and follow all the laws.

mother's loving care, he made little progress. It was becoming apparent that he might never walk again.

One summer day, his mother announced to him that, at her request, Miss Mary Baker Eddy, her Christian Science friend, was coming to heal Edgar's back. Although Edgar was skeptical, out of desperation he eventually agreed to have her try to help him.

Whether Miss Eddy had extraordinary powers or it was just Edgar's faith in his own healing powers, no one will ever know. However, shortly after her visit, he gradually began to regain his strength and eventually began to walk again.

During the summer of 1889, when Edgar was 17 years old, he started to feel much more like his old self. The question of what he was going to do with the rest of his life finally came up in a family council meeting.

In the discussion Edgar suggested to his parents that he might become a doctor. He had envied them during his multiple hospital stays. They seemed to have a good life and were treated with great respect.

Jennie emphatically disapproved: *"Your mother is a sincere believer in Christian Science, Edgar, and we don't believe in medicine. I will have no son of mine become a doctor of medicine."*

She continued, *"While you were away, I received a small legacy from England. I have some of the money left, and think it would be wise for me to spend it by taking you to New York, where we can get the advice of your Uncle John Parker, a successful business man."* Edgar liked his Uncle John and had much faith in his advice. Edgar's father agreed.

Uncle John was rather short and broad of beam, but he looked to be mostly muscle. He had the keen, penetrating eyes of an experienced seafaring man, which he had been before settling down on shore to become a ship chandler. He was a quick thinker and assertive in his speech and mannerisms. His mouth was firm and thin-lipped and looked as if it had been made by a horizontal cutlass slash. He sported mutton-chop whiskers, befitting of the time for a prosperous merchant.

Jennie Parker stated the sad case of young Edgar to Uncle John with all the gentleness she could muster, but it was still quite grim. Edgar was very uncomfortable as his mother disclosed all his sins of omission and commission. Jennie made it clear that Edgar was the despair of the Parker family. She summarized her feelings by saying, *"He's self-willed and no respecter of those in position, not even his own position as a member of the Parker family. His father has given up on him."* She then came right to the point: *"What can become of this boy's future? Edgar's physical condition prevents him from going back to the sea. We have come to ask you to help us set his feet on the right path. We feel a profession or a mercantile career would be a good selection for him. Could you not start him out in your ship-chandlery business as a bookkeeper or something like that until you find out what he is best suited for?"* Uncle John stroked his handsome beard and replied, *"Jennie, I feel for you. The problem is indeed a serious one. But I hardly think that a boy who has been five years sailing the before mast and has become acting second mate should be made into a bookkeeper! I am sure there must be something better for a lad like Edgar. Even though I might be able to use his seaman-ship training in my ship-chandlery business, I fear this industry doesn't hold a brilliant future. Sailing ships, which are the heart of my business, are becoming fewer and fewer as they are being replaced by this new fad of steam power. I'm not sure what will happen in the future, but one never knows."*

Uncle John pondered a moment, again pulling at his magnificent whiskers. Then, as if struck by an inspiration his face lit up, and he said, *"Why don't you have him phrenologized?"*

"What on earth is that?" Jennie asked. *"Is it painful?"*

"Oh, no," Uncle John reassured her. *"Phrenology is a science deter-mining the mental and occupational faculties by interpreting prominences on the skull. By feeling the bumps on Edgar's head, they can tell what Edgar is good for, what he can do best and in what occupation or profes-sion he will go the farthest. I recommend you take him to Professors Fowler and Wells, the famous phrenologists."*

Fowler and Wells had their flourishing business in an office located in what was then called "uptown," on East 27ᵗʰ Street. Edgar was taken into a booth and seated in a straight-backed chair. Then a man who looked to be about 80 years old and wore a black skull-cap shuffled in and began to feel the bumps on Edgar's skull. While the old man, whose name was Mr. Sizer, was feeling the bumps, he encouraged Edgar to talk about himself.

Another person, whom Edgar assumed to be Fowler, also came in and stood around. He studied Edgar intently, frowned and began making notes on a chart as Sizer called off the size and shapes of the various bumps.

"What's the boy's ambition?" Sizer asked Edgar's mother.

"He wants to be a doctor of medicine," she said, *"but I am a Chris-tian Scientist, and have strong feelings against this choice."*

Sizer scratched his chin and muttered, *"He seems to be okay to me, but there are a couple of stove bolts loose in his frame."*

Then Fowler spoke up, *"That's because he has an engine inside of him that's too big for his frame and he is shaking himself to pieces. Any-*

thing that this boy makes up his mind to do, you can depend upon it happening and being done well. His chart shows that he is outstanding along the mechanical lines and he cares about people's health. He rates well up in other lines, too: the scientific, commercial and professional. However, it all points to one thing. He would make a good dentist. Why not send him to dental college to study dentistry?"

Edgar remembered how the white-coated doctors in the hospitals had been respected. Being a dentist would be a good option considering his mother's aversion to medical doctors.

Edgar thought to himself, *"After only two years in college, I would have the title of Doctor, which should please my father, and maybe I could learn to be a good dentist and prevent other people from suffering with dental pain like my mother did."*

The next day, Edgar and his mother consulted Dr. Frank Abbott, the dean of the New York College of Dentistry, about enrolling Edgar for the fall term.

PRINCIPLE 28

If you want to gather honey, don't kick over the bee hive.

This is the best place to put Edgar's life on pause and discuss one more important principle that was revealed on his success path.

Most people choose a life path, and in dentistry, a practice type, by the "BE, DO, HAVE" method. However, truly successful individuals approach these decisions in a reverse order. Let me explain.

During school and on our way to adulthood we are frequently asked, *"What do you want to 'BE' when you grow up?"* Most of us don't have a clue.

My music teacher said I had lips for a trombone. He must have forgotten to look at the length of my arms.

My high school counselor told me I was good at math so I should be an engineer. At the time I didn't know an engineer, didn't know what they did and definitely didn't know what kind of money they made, yet I wasted one semester in college taking pre-engineering courses, before I had a revelation. Sound familiar?

We actually have a friend who decided to "BE" a speech pathologist. After graduating and working a year, she became disenchanted and went back to school to "BE" a speech pathologist with a master's degree. Twenty-five years later, at a class reunion she confided with us that she was unhappy with her career choices but felt trapped.

She didn't like what she had to "DO" as a speech pathologist. And she was certainly unhappy with her hours and remuneration, what she "HAD," but she felt trapped by all she had invested in her career.

As naive as Edgar's rationalization was, it was still on the right path. He decided he liked the "power and authority" that the doctors "HAD." He watched what they had to "DO" and figured he could do it. Even though he was slightly re-aligned into "Doctor of Dentistry" by his mother's discontentment for medicine, he settled into wanting to "BE" one.

The "Have, Do, Be" principle simply says you must first decide what is important to you. What do you want to "HAVE?" When you find folks who "HAVE" that, watch what they "DO" to get it. If you decide you could "DO" what they do, then determine what you will need to "BE" to get there.

We have all seen people who got into dental school because someone convinced them they needed to "BE" a dentist. But they later found out they didn't like anything a dentist had to "DO."

I have even witnessed dentists who say, *"I want to BE a 'cosmetic dentist.'"* They invest tens of thousands of dollars and more, travelling all over the place learning how to "DO" the work, only to find out that the practice they "HAD," after all was said and done, drove them nuts.

In my four decades of dentistry, I have seen several dentists who are what I call the "Shooting Stars." I see them touting themselves on TV as the "Cosmetic or Implant or Sedation Experts" one month, and high-tailing it out of town the next.

Wouldn't it be wiser to find someone who "Has" what you want: lifestyle, practice, income, etc., and then find out what they "DO" to create that? These individuals can make great mentors or coaches, even if you have to pay them. To list just a few of my mentors, Dr. Tom Orent, the Gems Guy, is my dental coach. Dan Kennedy is my business and marketing mentor. John Maxwell is my leadership and management mentor. Once you master what they "DO," you will "BECOME" someone like them. So now back to Edgar and his initial try at dentistry.

(Edgar and his mom at the dental college)

After they had talked with the dean, Jennie drew Edgar aside and told him that, after paying for the tuition and necessary books and instruments she would only have $200 left from her legacy for him to live on for the two years of college.

Edgar told her not to worry, that he would find a way to manage. He reminded her about how much money he had made while peddling from Moncton and finished with, *"I only need to find something that people want and I can sell it to them, even if I have to go door to door."*

At the New York College of Dentistry in 1889, Edgar studied the theoretical side of dentistry. Each student was assigned a preceptor to do the practical work. Edgar's preceptor taught him how to do laboratory work, like setting teeth for dentures, twisting dental gold to make bridges and casting gold to make inlays; however, when it came to patient care he was more reluctant.

Edgar's preceptor taught him how to clean teeth but wouldn't let him do extractions, fillings or other related dental services until he felt Edgar could clean teeth proficiently. His preceptor would pay him a small fee for cleaning the patient's teeth. But it was not enough for anyone to eke out an existence.

It wasn't long before Mrs. Parker's money legacy had run out. Edgar had to move in with Mrs. Maine, a friend of his mother's, who didn't charge him for the room.

After two days gaining experience at cleaning teeth for his preceptor, he decided to fall back on his New Brunswick peddling experience. Edgar chose to work mostly on 108th Street and on the West End Boulevard, which were considered one of the better districts out in the country. He went door to door and made $1 to $2 cleaning people's teeth. This provided him with enough money to keep going with food and personal needs.

When Edgar learned how to fill teeth, he carried a little dental hand drill and eventually provided cleanings, fillings and extractions in the living rooms and kitchens of the people's homes.

As Edgar told it, *"While the other boys were studying, I was getting enough to eat with my door-to-door dentistry. I carried my tools with me. I put my foot in a door and gave a spiel patterned after one I had I given as a peddler. I usually started with the cook's teeth. If I didn't kill the cook, and was lucky, I'd eventually wind up working on the teeth of the lady of the house.*

If I encountered problems that I hadn't yet come to in my dental-school education, I would postpone that treatment and return once we had covered that issue in class."

Before the college year was out, Edgar had opened his own office on the second floor at 17th and Broadway in New York City. It was 1890 and he was 19 years old. He placed a sign outside the building entrance. It readin large letters and beside his name there was a picture of a tooth. He hesitated to put "dentist" or call himself a doctor on the sign, as the New York dental laws were strict about that matter.

One day, a young Irish woman came into his office. She wanted gold restorations in her teeth. Edgar ran downstairs to Johnny Drennan, a salesman for the S.S. White Dental Company that was housed on the first floor. Drennan told Edgar how to place the restoration. Edgar started at 2:00 P.M. and finished at 2:00 A.M. He received $7 for his efforts, but it cost him $49 in gold. This lesson taught Edgar to project costs before quoting any prices for his service in the future.

Everything seemed to be working out very well. Edgar eventually learned to strike a delicate balance between classes and office work. Dr. Weisse, the professor of anatomy at the New York College of Dentistry, happened by Edgar's office building one day and noticed his sign. Upon further investigation, Dr. Weisse discovered that Edgar Randolph Rudolph Parker was one his students.

Edgar was called into the dean's office the very next day and was told by Dean Abbott that Dr. Weisse had informed him of Edgar's illegal dental activities. He said that it was a disgraceful situation and Edgar had placed the New York College of Dentistry in a most embarrassing and very awkward situation. If discovered, his activity could damage the school's excellent relationship with the dentists in the area.

Edgar was once again expelled from an educational institution. What was he going to do? Before answering that question, let me point out a few more success principles that Edgar learned in this episode of his life.

I'm not sure if Edgar initially knew what he had done but it was genius. He started his door-to-door dentistry in the more affluent areas. Things went well for him there for a couple of reasons. One, wealthy people have money to buy stuff. Even in down times wealthy people still have discretionary funds. The second reason is in principles 25 and 26.

Once Edgar made the cook happy he gained the rest of the household. That still works today. If you can provide a great dental experience to number one, they will lead you to numbers two, three and four.

Because Edgar was kind and courteous and provided good service to the cook, she would ultimately be the referral source to the lady of the house.

Think about it. If you treat someone special who is not used to it, even if they can't afford everything you have offered them, they are more taken aback than someone who is accustomed to first-class service. I can't tell you how many full mouth restoration cases I received from referrals of folks who could only afford an extraction.

The most valuable thing you can give someone is self worth. When you give someone that gift, the Law of Reciprocity kicks in and they immediately try to even the score. If folks leave your office feeling better about themselves, your office will never find itself running short of new patients.

This may sound dumb or even self evident, but there are many folks in all industries, including dentistry, who feel cheating or breaking the laws is the only way to get ahead. In the long run, that never works. In Edgar's case it worked for less than a year.

But in Edgar's defense, keep in mind what was going on in dentistry in 1890. The first dental school in the U.S. started in the mid 1800s. Most of the extractions were performed by physicians and barbers. By 1890, most of the schools were proprietary, non-affiliated with any formal university, and run as "for profit" organizations by the owners. The governing dental bodies at the time were either very loosely organized or non-existent in much of the United States and Canada.

The big reason Edgar was expelled from dental school had more to do with economics. The New York College of Dentistry would only work if the local dentists took on their students as preceptors. The school couldn't survive if the preceptor option was lost. If students were allowed to do dentistry on their own, local dentists could perceive the school's students as competition.

I'm not defending Edgar's judgment on this call, but you have to understand the context in which it was made. The way I see it, there are two types of dental violators. Those who are violating laws on purpose and those who are violating them and aren't aware of it.

The first group of dentists who commit insurance fraud, sell scripts or do something majorly stupid think that is the only way to make it, but they are dead wrong.

There are books, tapes, seminars and mentors that can open the doors to success for anyone if they are willing to learn and apply. I just wonder if they are too lazy or just don't know better.

When considering the second group of unaware violators, the story is much different. When I began practice in 1976 there was no OSHA or HIPAA and very few employment regulations. Today there are mountains of regulations and laws that are multiplying daily. This is why it is so hard for a solo private practitioner to keep up and abide by this rising tide of bureaucracy.

My warning to you is, unfortunately ignorance is never a good defense. If you are out there on your own, it is worth getting outside help in maintaining compliance.

Some punishment is severe enough to lose your license. In Edgar's case, he was fortunate enough to learn his lesson and eventually recover. Let's see how…

During the summer of 1890 Edgar borrowed an express wagon and mare from his grandfather and traveled throughout the rural districts of New Brunswick as an itinerant dentist.

There was hardly anyone in the province with a dental diploma. Dental laws were sketchy, if existent at all. As previously discussed, for the most part, extractions were performed by physicians and barbers with no formal training. Dental roots were typically left everywhere after an extraction.

As Edgar related later, *"After feeding my horse and paying board, I averaged $28 a day, all of which the noble profession of tooth fixers didn't like, but at that time my hunger was stronger than my ethics."*

By September 1890, he had saved enough money to pay for all his expenses for an entire year of study at a dental college. He decided to attend an institution where he could obtain a bona fide dental diploma. However, this time he vowed to be much more discreet if he did any dentistry off the college premises.

Edgar had heard from some of the students in New York that the Philadelphia Dental College (which eventually became Temple University) was a larger school and the dental students were able to carry out all phases of their dentistry at the college itself. Edgar preferred this to the preceptor model he had experienced at the New York College of Dentistry. He felt that the preceptor model tempted him into his last decision and he didn't want to be distracted again.

At the end of September, when he was 18, he set off for the Philadelphia Dental College to be, once again, enrolled in a two-year program.

The first year went well for Edgar. He lived in a boarding house and roomed with another dental student named Fred Seavers, from Minnesota. However, the second year presented problems financially and scholastically. He had nearly run out of money and needed to work again. He fell back on his door-to-door salesman methods, selling whatever became available. However, this time he did not try to sell dentistry. Consequently, he missed many lectures and barely made it through his exams.

When the notice of the spring commencement exercises for the class of 1892 was posted mid-February, it listed the names of the 142 students who would be receiving their dental diplomas. After casually reading through the list, Edgar re-read it more intently. His name was not on the list! This could not be right. Although he had just barely passed all of his examinations, he had passed. He was shocked. There must be a mistake!

He was filled with anger and his blue gray eyes sparked in rage. Edgar decided to immediately see the dean. When he went to the dean's office, Edgar was told that Dr. Garretson was at his home in Germantown.

Edgar Parker, the 20-year-old kid from the back woods of New Brunswick, only 5-foot-6-inches tall, decided to confront the dean, an impressive 6-foot-3-inch man, considered to be one of the greatest oral surgeons in the world.

Edgar found Dr. Garretson peacefully spading his garden. Edgar began the conversation angrily but cautiously, with great emotion in his voice, *"I'm surprised and disappointed not to be graduating."*

The Dean quietly replied, *"You really didn't expect to, did you?"*

Edgar sarcastically shot back, *"One doesn't get fat on expectations!"*

The dean responded softly and gently, *"You have missed some of my lectures, and that's inexcusable."*

Calming down somewhat, Edgar went on to build his case, *"Doctor, let me tell you the story of my life. It's been an uphill struggle all the way. As a teenager, I've been to sea, which is a tough life, even for a grown man. I came back from one trip so crippled that I am lucky to be walking today. For years, I have been earning my own way, peddling goods from house to house. I've had a tough life ever since I was a kid and I am sincere in asking if you would bend the petty rules just a bit and let me graduate. Rules don't mean much if you mean well when the chips are down."*

Dr. Garretson, obviously swayed by Edgar's forthrightness and sincerity relented, saying, *"All right, I'll take a chance on you, as long as you agree never to disgrace the College."*

So on May 28, 1892, Edgar Randolph Rudolph Parker received his dental diploma by the "skin of his teeth." Lets' examine one more important success principle before moving on to Edgar's next adventure as a Doctorate of Dental Surgery.

PRINCIPLE 29
Investigate the source of your information.

In this last episode, Edgar initially came attacking Dr. Garretson, and Garretson responded negatively. It wasn't until Edgar calmed down and tried a different approach that the dean finally softened and eventually allowed Parker to earn his dental diploma.

In his book, *How to Win Friends and Influence People* Carnegie shares a story about a sensational manhunt in New York City 1931 that climaxed on May 7, when "Two-Gun" Crowley was trapped in his sweetheart's apartment on West End Avenue.

Crowley, crouching behind an overstuffed chair, fired incessantly at the 150 policemen who had laid siege to his top- floor hideaway.

When Crowley was captured, Police Commissioner E.P. Mulrooney declared that the two-gun desperado was one of the most dangerous criminals ever encountered in the history of New York. *"He will kill,"* said the Commissioner, *"at the drop of a feather."*

But how did "Two-Gun" Crowley regard himself? While the police were firing into his apartment, he wrote a letter *"To Whom It May Concern, under my coat is a weary heart, but a kind one, one that would do nobody any harm."*

PRINCIPLE 30

Fear sells better than hope.

A short time before writing this note, Crowley had been caught necking with his girlfriend by a curious police officer. Without saying a word, Crowley drew his gun and began shooting.

When Crowley was sentenced to the electric chair and arrived at the death house he said to his observers, *"This is what I get for killing people?" "No,"* he said, *"This is what I get for defending myself."*

The point of the story is this: "Two-Gun" Crowley didn't blame himself for anything.

If "Two-Gun" and numerous men and women behind prison walls don't blame themselves for anything, what about the people with whom you and I come in contact every day?

Everyone feels they are right and telling them they are not doesn't change a thing. Instead of criticizing them, you can get much further by first trying to understand them.

I learned this Carnegie principle in the late 70s and have used the technique many times with staff, patients and even other dentists.

Another good source explaining this principle is Stephen Covey's book, *The Seven Habits of Highly Successful People*. Seek first to understand before attempting to be understood.

Chapter Thirteen

EDGAR RANDOLPH PARKER, D.D.S.

"Every sale has five basic obstacles: no need, no money, no hurry, no desire, no trust."

ZIG ZIGLAR

AFTER the graduation ceremony, Edgar immediately returned to his boarding house room, pulled out the yellow tin trunk from Scotland his mother had given him, sat down on top of it in front of his dresser mirror, stared at himself in the mirror and asked, *"Now Doctor, what next?"*

The answer came quickly, *"I will return home, practice in New Brunswick and show my father that his son, who at one time had horrified him by becoming a peddler, has at last brought honor to the Parker family name."*

Edgar gathered all his things, including his most valued belonging, his dental diploma, andheaded home to St. John. He was excited to show his parents his accomplishment. When he got home, he was not disappointed.

Soon after dinner on the first day of his return, George proudly introduced Edgar all around town. He bragged, *"My son, the doctor, is going to practice here."* Although it embarrassed Edgar a bit, his father meant well and was in his own way trying to drum up some dental business for his son.

PRINCIPLE 31

Preparation is critical.

Edgar's first impulse was to go out, like he did with his household items and almanacs and inform all these suffering uninformed inhabitants of the dental riches he had learned and brought back with him from Philadelphia. Then he suddenly remembered what he had been told so often at dental college: *"Never forget the 'dignity' of your profession."* This, of course, meant to solicit dental work in a direct fashion would be "unethical." It was fine to solicit work indirectly, by joining all of the clubs that were available, and never declining an invitation to be seen at any public place of entertainment.

"I would like to start a practice with dignity, but first I must have an office," Edgar muttered. *"Where?"*

The glory of being a freshly graduated dentist soon faded. Dr. Edgar Parker had counted on secur-

PRINCIPLE 32
Seeing is believing.

ing a loan from his father or one of the other Parker family members to open a somewhat pretentious establishment. However that never materialized. All he could borrow was his mother's sewing machine, which he rigged up as a dental lathe, and some portable screens that he could use as room dividers.

This didn't discourage Edgar. He was accustomed to fixing things and he did have all his hand instruments from dental school.

Edgar decided that St. Martins, the only place of any size near Tynemouth Creek, would be an ideal location to set up his practice. It had a shipbuilding industry, many stores and shops, and, most important, a number of wealthy people. He looked forward with anticipation to going back to his old home town where he had lived for three years, had attended high school and had gone to the seminary. His only concern was would the people of St. Martins remember all his boyhood escapades?

One of his old friends, who lived in St. Martins, had a house one block off Main Street. He agreed to let Edgar lease an L-shaped room there for $1 per month. With a place to live, Edgar was ready to find a place to open his practice.

After carefully surveying the downtown area, Edgar found several suitable locations that would work; however, when he inquired about them he was told there was nothing available that would serve his needs. Edgar got this uneasy feeling that many of the landlords weren't interested in having a dentist in their building.

He was told by a friend to check with Frank Bradshaw, the local barber, who did some tooth pulling when Dr. Henry E. Gilmore, the village physician and Edgar's uncle, was too busy. It was hinted that Frank had a two-chair barber shop with a spare chair and he might let Edgar use it.

Frank agreed to rent the space and the vacant chair to Edgar for $1 per month. Edgar arranged his mom's room dividers for privacy and added her rug and chairs to dress up his makeshift reception area.

Edgar placed his diploma in a conspicuous place on the office wall and sat down with great anticipation. After resolving the fact no one came, he concluded that he would need to try some other strategies to entice the apathetic patients in this village.

Edgar had been taught in dental college that the proper way to go after clientele was to join clubs. Because there weren't any men's clubs in St. Martins, he did the next best thing. He joined the church. He made it a point to attend religious services regularly in an attempt to get the people to know him. However, in spite of even these efforts, no one came.

Edgar thought that perhaps their hesitancy could have come from them remembering his shenanigans while at the Baptist seminary. So he decided to impress potential patients with his piety. He began to attend church twice each Sunday. He even strategized what pew would be more advantageous in accomplishing his goal. Still, no one came.

He wore his best clothes and carried the biggest Bible ever taken into the Baptist Church in St. Martins. Still, no one came.

Edgar volunteered for all the chores in the church, including passing the collection plate and singing the hymns louder than anyone else in the choir. Still no one came.

He assisted with services, taught Sunday school and did everything to make the people in the church think he was an ideal citizen. Still no one came.

Billy Woods, a sign maker in St. Martins, needed a new set of teeth. Edgar told Billy he would make him a new set of dentures in exchange for a sign. Billy agreed but on one term, that Edgar would make the dentures first. If Billy was happy, he would then paint a sign.

Edgar carried through on his promise and Billy was so pleased with his new teeth that he used an extra large slab of wood and painted in big lettering with gold leaf paint, Although Edgar was a little self conscious with its size, he was proud of his sign. To avoid any criticism he insisted it be hung after dark. That evening Billy nailed it up where it could easily be seen from the street corner. Edgar was certain that the next day, a line would form in front of his office.

He was wrong. Still no one came.

In fact, much to Edgar's distress, the very next night the sign was gone. He later found that someone had moved it to the town's train station outhouse door. After Edgar discovered it, he left it there all day because he didn't have the courage to take it down during the daylight hours in case someone might notice him doing it.

After returning the sign to its rightful place, it attracted only one patient over the next three months. The patient was a stranger passing through town with a terribly abscessed tooth. He noticed the sign and dropped in to see if Dr. Parker could help him. The tooth was so far gone that Edgar had to extract it. After the extraction, Edgar asked for a $1 fee. The stranger fished in his pocket and found only 75 cents. Edgar gratefully took it. Although it was not what Edgar wanted, he had finally serviced his very first, paying patient as a dentist.

When Edgar was speaking with George Mallory, a druggist and friend, about the lack of patients, his friend replied, *"Edgar, it's not that you got kicked out of Baptist seminary. It's nothing against you personally. It's just that people aren't accustomed to looking after their teeth and they are afraid of the dentist. They are afraid of getting hurt. If they don't have their teeth fixed, it's through ignorance, fear, lack of money or procrastination. If you want to affect a cure, you'll have to remove the cause."*

Those words stuck in Edgar's mind and eventually helped launch him on his future adventures. As he pondered what Mallory had said, he recalled reading some recent scientific papers about a new drug that could kill pain. It was so simple that he was flabbergasted that no one was routinely using it. The drug was called cocaine, and when it was injected into the gums it would numb them and the teeth in that area. Up until then, only general anesthetic had been used in dental offices. It didn't make much sense to Edgar to put someone to sleep just to do a filling.

He took the scientific paper to Mallory, who was also a chemist, and asked if he could make the cocaine combination deliverable by needle.

Mallory filled a crude horse syringe with the concoction and injected the recommended amount into a dog named Toby. The dog didn't bark, bite or die, so they concluded it must be safe to use on humans. Edgar called the mixture "hydrocaine."

He then injected a dose into Mallory's gums and, in turn, Mallory injected Edgar. Both experienced numbness and neither died. They even went on to make an incision in the numb areas and they still couldn't feel any sensation.

After 90 days, Edgar had tried everything he had been taught in dental college regarding how to attract patients, and he had only taken in 75 cents.

He recalled hearing of men who had used their title of "doctor" to acquire fortunes by marrying into wealthy families. So he tried it himself. In a single week he made three marriage proposals to different women from well-to-do families in St. Martins. Each time he was turned down because he had no visible means of support.

Edgar's father, George, was put out with Edgar's explanation about professional ethics. He told his son he was tired of being his "meal ticket" and that Edgar needed to get out and hunt for patients in the same manner that other business owners sought their customers. George was the first person Edgar had ever heard dispute the unrealistic dental college dictums about the ethical approach to building a dental practice.

After observing a Salvation Army captain delivering a fiery message in an open-air event and his Baptist minister do the same from the pulpit, Edgar realized that no one considered either of them as unethical.

Edgar began to formulate a plan. He started studying how to

speak publicly as he prepared a "sermon" of his own. His sermon would be about the horrifying bonfire awaiting the laggards who neglected their teeth. He memorized and rehearsed his speech so that he could complete it in 35 minutes without stopping. Edgar reasoned that if he could get a "congregation" to address, he could get some business. Once he had perfected his speech, he made the decision to go to a neighboring town and try it.

In early September 1892, he decided that the time had come. One morning, he abruptly announced, *"Mother, I'm leaving!"* Jennie Parker gave her son $25 to help clear his debts, so without a cent in his pocket and his dental gear in tow, Edgar hiked 25 miles away to a town called Hampton.

When he arrived, Edgar went to the Hotel Hampton and told the manager, *"I'm coming here to do some business and I need a room."*

"OK," replied the hotel owner.

Then Edgar borrowed a Baker Burner, a style of gas lantern used in those days, with a gasoline torch and 25 cents worth of fuel. He also borrowed a wagon that the hotel used to haul trunks and placed it in the street next to the hotel. He put up a pole with the lit Baker Burner fastened to it, tooted a dinner horn to attract a crowd and began his prepared talk.

He started from the back of the wagon. People began to gather and take notice to the light and the noise created by Edgar's speech. Eventually about 50 or 60 curious people had congregated around him. He lectured on the importance of keeping one's teeth clean and wound up with a climatic offer, *"I'll extract your bad tooth for only 50 cents, without hurting, using a new painkilling discovery."* He continued, *"But if you should experience any pain whatsoever at my hands, I will pay you a $5 bill. My friends, what could be any fairer than that?"* He elaborated at length about the amazing features of his new invention, hydrocaine. It seemed every other word Edgar uttered was "painless this and painless that."

During his talk a burly, unkempt heckler in the crowd shouted up to Edgar, *"Okay, you smart-aleck faker and so-called 'painless' dentist! Put your money where your mouth is."* Although Edgar didn't appreciate the interruption, it did give him an idea.

Maybe it wasn't a bad thing to be known as the 'painless' dentist. He could start referring to himself as Edgar Parker, the "Painless" Dentist, which over the years he eventually shortened to "Painless Parker."

At the same time, a little old fellow from a neighboring town came over and stood beside the back of the wagon. He had come to get a tooth pulled. After he clambered up onto the wagon and in the faint light of the gas burner, he said in a trembling voice, *"Mind you, Mister, if you hurt me, I'm going to yell."*

The tooth came out without incident. In fact, it was so painless that Edgar took out six or seven more for him right there on the spot. The crowd grew excited. Edgar took in $28 that night, with no refunds.

Using his earnings, Edgar was able to pay off all of his debts, including the one from his mother, and had money in his pocket to pay for his hotel room. He had made more money in one evening than he had earned over the preceding 90 days, sitting around waiting for patients to show up in St. Martins.

The next day he took in $20. Dr. Edgar Parker, the "Painless" Dentist, was officially launched. Edgar went out on the street every night, gave his speech and demonstration, and during the day, provide dental services in his make-shift hotel room-office. He stayed in Hampton for a couple of weeks.

During those two weeks, Edgar took in as much as $50 a day. In his mind he was rapidly becoming a professional success. Whether it was Edgar's father's disapproval about the lack of his success or his desire to educate about and help the poor unknowing crowds with their dental needs, it is uncertain what pushed Edgar into the street peddling once again. The one certain thing is that his future professional career would take a number of unexpected turns and twists. So let's pause before we explore his career any further and discuss a few more Parker Principles of success.

Edgar was advised not to advertise. He was told ethical dentists build their practices by joining clubs, being seen and waiting for patients to show up.

It always amazes me, when supposedly smart professionals who are taught to investigate the scientific resources before using a specific dental material in a patient's mouth, will take practice building advice from someone who probably doesn't have a clue what's happening.

In 1976, I was one of those supposedly smart professionals who made that same mistake. I was told to find out what the surrounding dentists in my practice area were doing and do what they did. So I worked the same hours, charged the same fees, provided the same services and advertised just like the other dentists in my community. Following that advice cost me 10 years of frustration and financial hardship.

This principle ties into the "Have, Do, Be" principle. If you want to have what a dental professor has, do what he does and you will be one. I'm not downgrading dental professors one bit. They do possess some things I don't, but they don't have a successful dental practice.

Dental school professors are great advisors on how to have an educational career, but that does not qualify them to dole out practice advice. If you violate this principle and do not investigate the source of your information, it could be expensive. It cost me 10 years.

There are mountains of books and articles written by thousands of authors on why people buy, and they all agree on one thing, people buy on emotion, not logic.

The emotions vary from self preservation, comfort, recognition, greed, convenience and fear, to mention a few. But what is strange, when it comes to these emotions, is that the fear of losing is much stronger than the opportunity to gain. The fear of losing comfort, self preservation and convenience motivates people to buy more often. I live in Oklahoma. When do you think storm cellars sell like hotcakes? Right after a tornado has ripped through the community. When do you think home security sales peak? Right after a burglary has happened in a given neighborhood. I could go on, but I think I have proven my point.

Edgar learned by watching a Salvation Army Captain and the St. Martins preacher that crowds were captivated by the fire and brimstone speeches warning the listeners what would happen to them if they refused to follow the advice given.

One of my mentors and coaches, Dr. Tom Orent, teaches a technique called "keel hauling." Keel hauling was the barbaric tradition captains used in olden days when they sensed that one of their sailors was about to cause a mutiny. The captain and those still loyal to him would bind the sailor's ankles, legs and hands; blindfold and gag the sailor and tie a rope to their ankles. They would then be thrown overboard from the old wooden ship while it was moving at full speed. They would drag the sailor underneath the keel of the boat along the sharp barnacles clinging to the bottom of the ship, and pull him back up the other side into the boat.

If the sailor died this technique was a great example and deterrent to the rest of the crew following such potentially mutinous behavior. Of course, if he lived, he was an even *better* example! Anyone who's heard that keel hauling story can't help but have a vivid graphic picture in their minds of this totally frightening, gory, heart-wrenching scenario. To "emotionally agitate" your patients requires that you put them into a similar emotional state. They must experience a *visceral* response to your description of their problem.

As I work with dentists on their case presentations, they typically spend too much time trying to logically sell the positives of crowning a tooth or replacing a space. They seldom stimulate the patients with what will happen if they don't follow the suggested course of action.

We equip them with stories that touch the patient's emotions; stories of patients who have neglected to deal with similar issues and the terrible outcomes they faced by doing so.

You seat yourself on an airplane headed for home. The pilot comes on over the cabin PA and says, *"Good morning, we are glad you have chosen to fly with us today. I'm not sure where we are going. I'll be firing up the engines soon and we will be up in the air before you know it. Once we are in the air, I'll wing it and see what happens."*

Would you start looking for the exit?

As absurd as this scenario sounds, dentists do this daily when presenting treatment plans.

Edgar was successful because he practiced his spiel until he had it down to the minute. My suggestion to all whom I coach is to develop your keel hauling stories—one or two for each type of treatment, then role play it over and over until it automatically slides off your tongue like boiled okra.

It is a good idea to choreograph your message in the same environment that you will be delivering it. It is also smart to video your presentation. Most social psychologists will tell you that nonverbal communication makes up about two-thirds of all communication between two people or between one speaker and a group of listeners. You can better evaluate your effectiveness if you can capture and perfect that two-thirds.

Parker's open-air demonstrations were eventually banned but when he was able to prove his painless pitch, his business exploded.

In today's digital world it shocks me how few dentists use this principle. Intra-oral cameras are cheap. Cell phones take OK pictures of happy patients and can capture audio testimonies. Remember, patients buy just like everyone else, from emotion. How impactful is seeing someone else who was in a similar circumstance triumphantly making it through to the other side?

Chapter Fourteen

THE FIRST MOBILE DENTIST
WAS LAUNCHED

"Action is the foundational key to all success."

PABLO PICASSO

IT became increasingly clear to Edgar that trying to establish himself as a "dignified" dentist in rural New Brunswick was hopeless. He didn't have enough money to hold out while he waited for patients to appear, and he couldn't sponge off his father forever. He had tasted the excitement of street dentistry and appreciated the quick money it brought. He had grown to like being a salesman and dentist at the same time.

The big problem that now faced Edgar was how he was going to earn a living. He thought of Horace Greely's advice: *"Go west, young man!"*

One weekend while he was in Hampton, he went to St. John to see Jack Kirkpatrick, a friend from his Acadia College days. At that time, Jack was working as a clerk in Gilbert's Furniture and Carpet Store. Jack's experience there had taught him how to meet people and sell his product.

"Let's go west, Jack," Edgar said to him, *"Let's start out together and find a place where we can grow up with the country, where they won't hold you back because you are young."*

"I'd gladly go with you, Edgar," Jack replied with a bit of hesitation in his voice, *"but let's face it, it takes money. How will we get the money to travel west?"*

"We don't need much," answered Edgar, *"only enough to get to the first town. I have a great idea! I used to make money selling almanacs and notions to farmers and other items to city folks. Anything that people need they will buy if you go to them and tell them about it, even if at first they think they can't afford it.*

I have something people need very much. That is dental care. I can make my prices low enough that almost anyone can afford it. You can promote our business by distributing the handbills that will tell the towns-people about my services. You can also be my assistant and help me deliver the care and do some of my lab work. I can teach you all you need to know. We can divide the pot."

Edgar's argument convinced Jack to give it a try.

"I have a little money put back," said Jack, *"enough to get us started. But I'll hold out enough for a return ticket just in case it doesn't work out."*

Edgar then went home to talk it over with his parents. As expected, his father was against the plan.

"It is not dignified for you to go out and peddle your dentistry," Edgar's father said. *"It's not in keeping with a professional man. What will people think?"*

Edgar's mother spoke up: *"It makes no difference what other people think so long as what Edgar wants to do is honest."*

Edgar clung to his mother's words for the rest of his life.

Jack and Edgar were both 20 years old when they headed 600 miles northwest of St. John to Montreal on September 15, 1892. They both thought it was a perfect big city in which to launch their new business venture. However, there was one problem.

After taking account of all their available resources, they discovered they didn't have enough to buy two train tickets to get there. So they altered their original plan. They decided to stop in small communities along the way, make some money and then continue westward until they finally reached Montreal.

The first target was Vanceboro, a small railroad town in the northern tip of Maine. Once they reached Vanceboro, they rented a hotel room. Jack started distributing flyers announcing the arrival of "Dr. Edgar R. Parker, Dentist," while Edgar converted the hotel room into a suitable dental office.

Edgar had a portable dental engine that he had used while in dental college. It operated by foot and was light enough to carry under his arm. He also had a satchel of instruments and bottles containing various antiseptics and medications. He set up his drill and instruments on clean towels strewn across a table.

He used an ordinary rocking chair borrowed from the hotel's front porch as a dental chair. He placed the rocking chair on a soapbox he borrowed from the kitchen to raise and steady it. He placed another soapbox in front of the chair to be used as a footrest.

PRINCIPLE 33

It's not how many times you go down that counts. It is how many times you get up.

Edgar was ready to practice dentistry. He waited for patients to come in. The numbers started slow and dried up totally by the fourth day, so Edgar and Jack decided it was time to go.

When they tallied what they had made, it wasn't much. But it was enough to pay for the hotel room and two train tickets to the next stop, Jackman, Maine. This time they approached their business model a bit differently.

After Jack had distributed the circulars, Edgar had him stay at the hotel to meet the patients and schedule them for Edgar's return. Edgar went door to door, telling the residents that he was passing through town and he was prepared to do their dentistry at the local hotel.

Edgar found the townspeople very friendly and they seemed pleased to have someone explain dental issues to them. He realized that going out to the people in their own homes helped generate more interest and business.

They stayed in Jackman for nearly a week. After Jack had paid all the bills, they were pleasantly surprised with their $100 profit.

They felt like plutocrats! Jack and Edgar bought three bottles of whisky and shared their good fortune with the train crew between Le Megantic and Montreal. The crew became so drunk that Jack had to run the engine while Edgar ran the caboose. Edgar was sure they would go off the tracks at any moment, but finally the crew sobered up enough to finish the trip into Montreal. Edgar and Jack were living large on the $100 they had earned by the time they arrived in Montreal.

Although Montreal was a large city with a European feel, it threw a slight kink in their marketing model. Most of the folks in Montreal spoke French. So the flyers and Edgar's door-to-door visits wouldn't work.

PRINCIPLE 34

You can gather a crowd quicker when you have an enemy.

While in Montreal, they met a young man named Harry Crosby. Crosby had previously worked in a dental laboratory and knew how to make plates, bridges and many other dental appliances. He told them that he had also worked as a dentist, but he didn't have a diploma or a license to practice.

Crosby informed Edgar that his diploma from a first-class American dental college wouldn't permit him to practice dentistry in Montreal. The local dental association had recently passed an exclusionary law requiring a special examination with a substantial fee to acquire a license to practice dentistry in Montreal. And as it were, the examination wouldn't be given again for several months. Edgar was pretty sure they would run out of money before then.

Edgar asked Cosby if the examination would be hard.

"Not at all," replied Cosby. *"It's just a formality. The real idea is to make it difficult, if not impossible, for untrained or outside dentists to come to Montreal to practice. Local dentists wanted to restrict competition from 'outside' dentists. No matter how good you are, no matter how many diplomas you have, there is a $250-a-day penalty if you are caught practicing in Montreal without a local license. It looks as if you are out of business here, Edgar."*

Edgar was shocked! He had never heard of such a thing as a group of professionals banding together to bar outsiders. It seemed to be so unfair and undignified!

To test the rumor, he called on some Montreal dentists, showing them his diploma and telling them he was thinking about setting up practice in their beautiful city. He soon found out Crosby was right.

For the most part Edgar was not welcomed by the Montreal dentists. One actually told him, *"You'd better get out of Montreal and find some other place where dentistry isn't so well organized."*

While visiting J. Carlos McLean, D.D.S., a dentist located in Beaver Hill, an exclusive area of Montreal, Edgar helped himself to some of Dr. McLean's business cards that were in the reception area. Edgar thought, *"One can never tell when one of these cards may come in handy."*

By this time, Jack and Edgar had already spent almost a week in Montreal at the expensive Windsor Hotel. They soon realized they had only 11 cents left from their Jackman purse, which wouldn't be enough money to pay their hotel bill, due in three days.

After Crosby had heard how Jack and Edgar had made it to Montreal, he encouraged them to continue. *"That's a swell idea!"* Cosby remarked. *"Let's work together as a team. I'd like to go with you. Jack can travel ahead distributing the circulars and announcing that 'Doctor Edgar R. Parker and Staff' are coming. Then he can join us when we arrive and act as our receptionist. I'm a good lab man. You can do twice the dentistry if you have me along. I can make plates, crowns and bridges after you take the impressions. We can go west through the province of Ontario. I don't think they have any dental license laws there, yet. What do you say?"*

Jack thought it was a fine idea, and Edgar agreed. The partnership formed, they opened a Canadian Pacific Railroad folder and again looked for towns along the line. Chalk River, Ontario was the next targeted town.

However, their idle conversation didn't bring them any money, which is what they desperately needed.

Edgar, not wanting to get in trouble with the Montreal law, needed cash quickly. He sold six bottles of hydrocaine to Patterson & Foster dental supply. With that money he purchased a Canadian Pacific Railroad ticket to the nearest town outside Montreal, Hochelaga.

Edgar carried his portable dental engine under one arm and a satchel of instruments under the other. He felt reasonably certain he was safe from the Montreal dental laws in Hochelaga.

An older woman in the third house Edgar visited expressed a need for dental work. However, she had no money to pay for it. He worked out a deal to swap her dental work for three days boarding in her rather large home. Both were satisfied with the deal.

Edgar discovered going door to door doing dental work right in the homes of his patients worked reasonably well. At the end of three days he sent enough money to Jack to pay the hotel bill, allowing him to move to a cheaper one.

Edgar's landlady suggested he go to St. Remi, a town 20 miles south of Montreal. She said there was a big Catholic convention going on and people would be visiting from miles around.

Edgar made his way to St. Remi and found the town bustling, with gaily dressed men and women filling the sidewalks and streets. However, there was again one big drawback: everybody in town spoke French, except that is, Edgar.

Struggling with the language barrier Edgar finally negotiated a room at the Gatineau Hotel.

He sauntered down the main street, wondering how he could inform these people that he was a dentist ready, willing and able to fix their teeth. Suddenly he noticed a bright-looking, dark-eyed man parading down the avenue, stopping occasionally to loudly proclaim something he had written on a printed sheet of paper in French. Edgar thought, "That fellow could be a real asset to me if I could get him to tell the people that the 'painless' dentist was in town ready to receive patients."

When Edgar approached the man, he was surprised to be spoken to in English: *"I am Jean Berthier, the town crier. I see that you are a stranger in St. Remi. Can I be of assistance to you?"*

"Yes," replied Edgar, giving him a business card that he had retrieved earlier in Montreal, *"my name is J. Carlos McLean, the noted Montreal dentist. I am in town for a few days and would like to help the people in this community with their dental needs. However, I don't speak French."*

"That is unfortunate," Berthier said courteously. *"May I translate for you? My fees are low."*

"Let's go over to the Gatineau Hotel and discuss the possibilities," Edgar proposed excitedly. *"I have a proposition to make."*

After Edgar showed Berthier his dental setup at the hotel he explained, *"I'd like to hire you to announce in French that Dr. J. Carlos McLean, the renowned Montreal dentist, is here to care for their teeth, without any pain or waiting, at the Gatineau Hotel. If anyone has any questions about who I am, just give them my business card."* With that he gave Berthier a handful of Dr. McLean's business cards.

"Certainly," answered Berthier, *"I'll do it for a modest fee of, let's say, 10% of what you bring in."*

Edgar agreed.

"Ah, yes, but first, Dr. McLean, before I do my job, you must make a demonstration," Berthier said.

"A demonstration! What do you mean by a demonstration?"

"Could you pull a few teeth in public?" Berthier asked cautiously.

"Oh, to be sure!" Edgar responded smartly, *"I can pull teeth anywhere there are people with teeth and as long as they want them pulled. I've done it many times before."*

"Follow me," said the town crier. He tucked Edgar's portable dental machine under one arm, grabbed a chair from the hotel porch with the other and led the way to a tiny park-like space in the center of a crowded street only a short distance away. Edgar quickly got the idea and set up his foot-powered dental drill.

A curious crowd quickly gathered to watch the proceedings with mounting interest. Then Berthier began to speak to them in French. As he spoke, his voice became louder, more excited and increasingly animated. Then he began to wave his arms wildly, motioning toward the chair.

Soon a man came from the crowd, sat in the chair and pointed to a tooth. Edgar recognized the offending tooth immediately; it was so lose that it was almost ready to fall out. He extracted it so deftly and quickly that the man didn't feel anything. The patient smiled broadly as Edgar showed him the tooth in his raised forceps. What an impressive demonstration!

The town crier grabbed Edgar's hand, still clutching the blood-covered tooth in the forceps, and held it even higher in the air.

Edgar didn't know what Berthier told that crowd, but from his expressive gestures and eloquent facial expressions, Edgar was certain that he must have told them that this dentist was just shy of a miracle worker!

The man handed Edgar 50 cents and cleared the way for another anxiously standing behind. He also had a lose tooth that needed extracting.

In a few minutes, the town crier turned to Edgar and said, *"No more here. Pack your satchel, and we will lead this crowd to your hotel room."*

Berthier grabbed the chair and dental engine, Edgar picked up the dental instruments and the entire entourage, chattering loudly, started back to the Gatineau Hotel.

Edgar set up the equipment in his room while the town crier led patients into the room one by one. Occasionally, Edgar could hear the comforting sound of Berthier delivering his oration on the street in front of the hotel.

Each time he returned from his talk, he was followed by another group of patients. The town crier was a genius! After two days, the convention in town had ended. Edgar paid Berthier his 10%, paid the hotel bill and still had $86 profit.

Then things took an unexpected turn. Edgar was called on by a dentist who lived in St. Remi. From the look on the visitor's face, Edgar knew that it wasn't just a social call.

The town crier translated, *"This man, our local dentist, says he wants to see your Quebec license."*

Surprised, Edgar asked, *"What license? Isn't Montreal the only place you need a license? I have a diploma, but my license is back in Montreal."*

The two talked further in French, then the local dentist stormed out.

"I told him that you had left your license in Montreal," explained Jean Berthier, *"and you will wire for it and expect to have it tomorrow."*

He looked sympathetically at Edgar's crestfallen face. *"If you do* not have a dental license in Quebec," he said, trying to be helpful, "my advice is that you not be here tomorrow, my friend. Without a license, your diploma is not valid. The license law is for the entire province of Quebec. The fine for violating this law is $250 a day! He said he would be back tomorrow with the authorities to check out your story."

Edgar took the town crier's advice to heart. He left early the next morning right after sending Jack this telegram. "The dental license law applies to the entire province of Quebec. We've got to get out of here, quick! You and Crosby meet me in Chalk River tonight."

Once in Ontario, they found laws similar to that of Quebec. The bright spot was they had discovered a dental diploma was all that was necessary in Michigan. After barely squeaking out an existence for the three of them in Sault Ste. Marie and Gladstone, Michigan, the partnership started to unravel.

Edgar had a heart-to-heart talk with Jack and Crosby. He told them there wasn't enough dental business in the Gladstone area and that he wanted to go further west. Crosby got angry and informed Edgar that he had had enough and was heading back to Montreal. Jack said he had seen all he wanted to see of the west and would be returning to St. John. The partnership broke up that day. Edgar took his share and moved on to St. Paul-Minneapolis, Minnesota.

In 1892, St. Paul was a booming business center. In Minneapolis, just a few miles up the Mississippi, the growth was even larger. While Edgar was scoping out the area, he was suddenly attacked by three men. Edgar struggled to get free but soon realized they had taken his money in the scuffle. He had been set up! Edgar still had his wallet with his train tickets and a single dime in his pocket. He went through his upper vest pocket and found a folded $2 bill.

When he returned to his hotel he pled his case to the clerk, who remained unmoved. The clerk told Edgar that he could take his handbag, but the hotel would have to keep his trunk as security until his hotel bill was paid. Although Edgar protested vigorously, the manager's mind was made up.

There was nothing left for Edgar to do, so he climbed aboard a long Northern Pacific tourist train to Tacoma, Washington, with only $2 in his pocket to pay for all his meals for the next six days. To his chagrin, he was leaving behind his most prized possession, his dental diploma, which was held captive by the hotel manager.

Fortunately, Edgar had purchased his train tickets before the partnership had ended. At that time he had enough money to buy first-class coach fare.

The first class coaches were made up into bunks, with a stove on one end of the car for warmth. Most of the people on the tourist cars traveling west carried their own food.

There he was, all dressed up like a Mississippi River gambler wearing a fine hat and coat. It wasn't obvious to anyone that he had only $2 to his name.

Edgar even thought about trying to meet some of the eligible women on the train. In doing so, he discovered that by making conversation with nicely dressed folks who had tin washboilers, (containers used to store food), he was eventually invited to share their provisions.

Over the next six days, Edgar refined this approach to the point where he arrived in Tacoma with the $2 still in his possession. He never had to spend a penny.

But, by the time he checked into a hotel in Tacoma and bought a couple of meals, he was again down to his last 2 cents. Edgar realized he needed some quick cash. Once again he gathered his dental equipment and went house to house. The people in Tacoma seemed to be freer with their money, so this enabled Edgar to charge fees several times higher than he had ever received before. Later that evening he came back with $28.

The next day on a busy main street, Edgar noticed a neat sign on a second floor building. It read "Manly C. Burns D.D.S." Edgar knew him well! He had been the valedictorian of the class ahead of Edgar at the New York College of Dentistry. Edgar called on him. At first Dr. Burns was glad to see him. But when Edgar started sharing his financial plight, Burns hastily explained that he was to be married soon and had no spare money to loan his classmate.

When Edgar told Dr. Burns he thought that Tacoma would be a fine place for him to open a practice also, Burns responded quickly, *"You can't practice in the state of Washington without a license. That re-*

quires a test that will not be given for another six months."

"That damn dental-monopoly law again! It's designed to keep newcomers out!" exclaimed Edgar. Realizing Dr. Burns wasn't much of a friend, he once again travelled house to house out in the country. There he provided dental care and came back with $45 in his pocket.

Since his hotel room was costing him $10 a day, Edgar decided it was time to move on. The next day he went to the nearest ferry ticket office and used his last dollar to buy a ticket on the Oregon Railway and Navigation Company's line of steamers direct from Tacoma to Vancouver, British Columbia. He was broke again!

Edgar was able to make contact with some relatives on a three-hour stopover on the way to Vancouver in Victoria, British Columbia. After hunting up George Meldrum, George did remember some relatives named Parker from Tynemouth Creek, New Brunswick. On his short visit with them, Edgar graciously accepted a free meal, since peanuts were all he had eaten since commencing his ferry trip.

As soon as he arrived in Vancouver, Edgar hustled from house to house with his dental kit to raise a little money. Vancouver was not as prosperous as he had been led to believe. He took in enough to get himself back to Victoria on the next ferry, with only a few dollars left over.

Edgar decided Victoria would be a better place for him. It was safer than Vancouver and he knew he could wrangle some of Mrs. Meldrum's splendid home-cooked meals once in awhile.

His relatives persuaded Edgar to set up a dental practice in Victoria. Almost immediately he was able to secure temporary work with Dr. W.J. Quilan, who wanted to take a two-month vacation to Alaska. Quinlan told Edgar that he would fix it with the dental board so that Edgar could practice until his diploma arrived. Edgar was to operate his office, on a percentage basis, while Quinlan was away. Edgar would pay 25% of all he made to Quinlan to cover the rent and other expenses. He would be able to keep the rest. Life was good during those two months. After he had paid his bill at the hotel in St. Paul to retrieve the trunk with his diploma, Edgar was able to save some money.

He continued his working relationship with Quinlan several

months after Quinlan returned from Alaska. Edgar used those earnings to pay rent for an office of his own and also purchased some dental equipment. However, after paying for a sign, some business cards and some announcements, he was broke again.

Much to his disappointment, Edgar learned the hard way that British Columbia also had a dental license law. While working with Dr. Quinlan everything seemed to be fine, but the second he started his own practice, things changed. Soon after he had sent out his opening announcements, an inspector from the dental board called on Edgar and demanded the $25 license fee. Not having the money at the time, Edgar tried unsuccessfully to postpone his payment for a day or two. Dr. Quinlan had said he would loan Edgar the money for the license, but happened to be out of town for a few days when the inspector arrived.

On his 21st birthday, Edgar was admiring his new office and sign in Victoria, when his first patient arrived. The stranger asked, *"Are you Dr. Parker?"*

Edgar answered, *"Most assuredly, sir."*

The man said he was going out to the Bering Sea in a few hours on a seal hunting trip. He begged Edgar to fix his teeth before going to sea, as he was suffering much misery. Edgar felt the humanitarian thing to do was to help the gentleman. So he prepared his office to do the work. After a preliminary examination, Edgar was surprised when he couldn't find anything wrong with the stranger's teeth. Although Edgar was a bit suspicious, the stranger begged him to do something.

Edgar cleaned the man's teeth with a scaler, hoping that it would bring relief. The patient rose from the chair all smiles. He thanked Edgar and said the pain was gone. Edgar was somewhat perplexed because he felt he had done nothing that would have really helped the pain. The seaman appeared grateful as he handed Edgar a $5 bill, which Edgar stuffed in his pocket.

Suddenly the stranger flashed a badge and told Edgar he was under arrest for practicing dentistry without a license. He proceeded to tell Edgar that he had been hired by Dr. T.J. Jones, the secretary of the dental association, as a "spotter" to catch Parker practicing dentistry without a license. Edgar had again been set up!

Edgar's first impulse was to protest, but he knew that under Canadian law, resisting an officer was a serious offense. Then he saw his new sign on the shelf behind the spotter's head. An idea came to him. He casually walked over to the unused sign, picked it up and gave the officer a sufficient whack on the head to knock him out. Edgar bent down, put the $5 back into the imposter's pocket, meekly walked down to the police station and turned himself in.

As luck would have it, while Edgar was being booked, he discovered that the Chief of Police was a Meldrum, a relative on his mother's side. The Chief had learned what was going on and said, *"Young Parker is a cousin of mine. I will personally go his bail."* The chief told Edgar to see the judge. The judge lent Edgar $100 and told him to use $25 of it to register his diploma and get a dental license.

Once he had followed the judge's instructions, Edgar went to Dr. T.J. Jones' office. There he stood up and loudly shouted, in his best peddling voice, for people passing to stop and listen to him because he had something very important to tell them.

A crowd quickly gathered and Edgar told them exactly how he had been set up by Dr. T.J. Jones. He explained that Jones knew he had a diploma and nothing was said about him practicing dentistry in Victoria until he had opened his own practice and threatened Jones with some competition.

"That's why he set me up," yelled Edgar. Soon the people in the audience began to hiss every time Dr. T.J. Jones' name was mentioned.

With his $25 license and registration certificate posted on the wall, Edgar opened his office again early the next morning.

Word spread like wildfire about this brash, gusty new dentist in town. Patients thronged to his office all day long. Canadian laws might be strict, but Canadians had a strong sense of fairness. Thereafter, Dr. Jones' practice dwindled, as Edgar's dental practice thrived.

When the case against Edgar was called in court, neither Dr. Jones nor the "spotter" appeared, so it was dismissed.

Before forging on, let's step back a moment and glean a few

more principles of success learned from this segment of Edgar's life.

OK, so let's be truthful. How many times did it go through your mind while reading this episode of Edgar's life, *"Enough is enough. Surely Edgar will retreat here."?*

How many times could you have handled being run out of town due to a non-compete law? How many times could you take being flat broke before throwing in the towel? What about when Jack and Parker left and he was faced with going it alone?

I remember the night I learned this principle. It was a spring evening in 1987, while I was visiting a friend and mentor, Robert Echols, in Longview, Texas. After arriving at his home that afternoon and having a great meal that evening, we retired to his living room. I started to share my despair.

PRINCIPLE 35

One is the worst number in business.

"It's just not fair Robert. "I whined. *"I have spent 10 years working my butt off and have nothing to show for it and now I lose a son. I'm not sure it's all worth it."*

Robert listened intently and empathetically then said, *"Kelly, let's go outside and get a bit of this East Texas Spring air."*

I obliged and headed out onto the porch just as the sun was setting, and the sky looked as if it were on fire.

As soon as we were outside Robert strolled over and grabbed a wash cloth that was on top of his outside grill. He then bent over and with the other hand picked up an old tennis ball that the dogs had used as a toy.

He looked me dead in the eye and threw the ball and the wash cloth directly down onto the concrete floor and said, *"Kelly, life is not fair. As a matter of fact from time to time it will slam you to ground. Many times you will not have a choice on when or how it happens. But you will have a choice on how you will respond. Will you splat like that wash cloth or will you rebound like that tennis ball? The decision is yours. And always remember, your family's future will be forever affected by that decision."*

So, when a critical staff person leaves, or your office faces a major setback, remember W.W.P.P.D. *"What would Painless Parker do?"* And make the decision, *"Will I be a wash cloth or a tennis ball?"*

This is a very important marketing principle that I see few dentists employing.

I'm not sure whether Edgar was blowing off steam, getting revenge or was aware of this principle, but it worked. He inspired his audience into action when he painted Jones as the villain. This ultimately gave him momentum in his own practice.

I wouldn't recommend thrashing your competitor dentists or taking your cause to the street to gather a crowd. However, there are numerous causes that can stir the emotions of certain folks in your community like: neglected pets, battered women, homeless children, families afflicted with a debilitating illness, breast cancer... The list goes on.

At Custom Dental, we use these causes for promotional events, direct mail pieces and image building. We have supported fire departments that were facing funding cuts, animal shelters that had burned

PRINCIPLE 36

You can learn something from everyone.

down, families who had lost homes in tornados, Relay for Life events that raise breast cancer awareness and many other causes. Using this principle draws crowds, creates emotional ties and can spawn lifetime loyalty within your practice.

Chapter Fifteen

PARKER WANDERLUST CONTINUES

"Without promotion something terrible happens...Nothing!"

P.T. BARNUM

IT was October 1893, and 21-year-old Edgar, having practiced his trade in Victoria for almost a full year, believed that he was due a break from "fixed" dentistry. He had accomplished one of his goals of providing dental services in one stable location.

However, he began to realize this style of practice didn't meet his expectations.

PRINCIPLE 37

If you don't toot your own horn, you may never be heard.

Edgar felt that the typical practice of dentistry was very inefficient and restrictive. He had only one pair of hands and only so much time. True, they were highly skilled hands, but he couldn't make money unless they were actually producing dentistry. He found that the business of dentistry consumed much of his time, but brought in no income.

It all boiled down to the fact that any single-handed person could only provide good dentistry at a high cost. He believed that the solo-dentist method was an unproductive luxury.

Although Edgar had some ideas on how to improve things, he knew it would take more capital than he had. He also realized that with this radical departure from the norm, he would face some major opposition from other dentists and dental organizations. It was a plan he knew would work but the timing wasn't yet right for him.

He thought to himself, *"One of these days, my time will come."* How prophetic that was!

After returning from a seal-hunting trip at the end of November 1893, Edgar heard about a dental job working for the Alaskan Territorial government. They paid $125 a month. He thought taking care of Indian and Eskimo teeth in Sitka, Alaska, would be a great adventure. With his room and board covered, the $125 a month would be more than he was making after expenses in Victoria. He applied for the job, and he got it!

He sold his practice in Victoria with all of its equipment and contents, except for his faithful portable dental kit. It had proven a blessing in the past and Edgar knew, if times got tough, he could always fall back on what he knew, house-to-house dentistry.

Sitka was the Alaskan Territorial capital. Its population was about 150, most of whom were Indians and Eskimos. Eking out a living trading with the local Indians was a tough life and, other than government officials, there were few other whites in Sitka.

The climate was terrible. It was not so much the cold as it was the penetrating moisture of the rain and fog that brought in over 80 inches of rain per year.

Although the famous Alaskan-Yukon gold rush didn't happen until 1896, some gold was being found in Sitka in 1893. This meant miners were starting to infiltrate the soggy community. Following them were saloons and floozies.

Edgar continued to dress like a Mississippi River boat gambler—in his long, fancy coats and a tall top hat that made him a target for many of the chorus girls and jealous, drunk miners. That winter he sustained several facial scars and two bullet holes in his hat. Edgar felt lucky to be alive.

When spring came, the sap started rising in the trees, and also in Edgar. He realized that he was still a young man, full of health and optimism. He was a man with a vision. He felt destined to bring tooth salvation to millions and Sitka was not the place to launch his mission.

On the day he appeared at the Sitka docks to catch the first spring ship south to Seattle, all he had to show for his winter work were two bullet holes in his top hat.

In Seattle, Edgar was not surprised to find out that he would have to wait many months for the next state dental board examination to be given.

While he was in a hotel lobby one afternoon in April 1894, he happened to meet a large-framed, formidable-looking man dressed in a black frock coat. He wore a broad-brimmed black sombrero hat atop a thatch of glossy, dark, shoulder-length hair. Although he had an air that would make some feel threatened, Edgar soon found himself confiding in the gentlemen about his struggles trying to make a living as a dentist.

"Young man," he said, *"I think I can teach you some things that will help you along the road to fame and fortune. How would you like to travel with me and wear diamonds?"*

"But, I don't even know your name," Edgar said, somewhat taken back by the stranger's forward manner. *"And if I should travel with you, what would you have me do?"*

PRINCIPLE 38

People will pay for what they want.

"How rude of me! First, permit me to introduce myself." The tall stranger replied with self importance and confidence. *"My name is William True. The Great William True!"*

"You are very modest." Edgar sarcastically replied.

"No!" retorted True, *"I am not modest! But, sir, I detect a bit of sarcasm on your part that, in my opinion, could be a sign of stupidity. This concerns me because if you are stupid, I hesitate to invite you to come with me."*

Edgar sat up with a jolt. It was the first time anyone had ever blatantly called him stupid to his face. Those were fighting words.

"What do you mean?" Edgar shouted back while clenching his fists.

"I mean a little personal modesty is all right, but too much modesty in one's business or profession is stupidity," William True replied calmly.

"Remember this: If you don't toot your own horn, more than likely no one will do it for you."

With a bow, he handed Edgar his card. It read:

THE GREAT WILLIAM TRUE

Lecturer, Scholar, Teacher – Adept in
Psychology And Magician

Discover the Extraordinary Marvels of

TRUE'S MEDICINAL MINERAL SALTS!

"You are a patent-medicine man!" gasped Edgar, as he read the card. Edgar had been warned about such quacks while at dental college.

"Correct," said True. *"But more importantly, I can teach you how to toot your own horn and how to handle large crowds of people. All of this will help you bring more patients for treatment than you can ever imagine in your wildest dreams."*

Edgar began to reminisce about his frustrating interactions with crowds while peddling his almanacs and outdoor dental shows. He thought, *"This stranger might be an egomaniac, but he sure is making sense!"*

"Put on your hat and come with me," directed True as he led the way to a nearby livery stable. There he showed Edgar his wagon. On the outside it looked similar to the one which Edgar had when he peddled almanacs in New Brunswick as a 15-year old-kid. However, it was larger and heavier and had a removable canvas top that made it resemble a schooner.

PRINCIPLE 39

Collections do not equal profits.

True climbed onto the wagon, flipped down various panels, lifted the top of one of the seats and revealed to Edgar's astonished eyes a self-contained operation, complete with bunks and a stove. Next, True closed the panels, replaced the lids, lowered the canvas top and hung up a Baker gasoline torch. And behold! It was now an attractive stage, bright with new paint and perfect for performing open-air shows.

Edgar was both impressed and fascinated.

In a nearby stall, True showed Edgar two big shiny horses that were used to pull the wagon. They resembled the one he had in New Brunswick.

Finally, True introduced Edgar to "George Washington," a 200-pound black man who had a smile as broad as the Bay of Fundy. "Wash," as True called him, played the banjo in the medicine show, sang melodies, cooked the meals and took care of the horses.

As Edgar sampled Wash's delicious green-apple pie, he recalled the awful Siwash food he had endured all winter in Alaska. The pie was delicious.

True seemed to be weaving a magic spell over Edgar as he started mentoring him on the ways of the medicine show and what he needed to do to learn the "pitch." Their next pitch would be in a town called Black Diamond, Washington.

True rented a vacant lot on the main street in Black Diamond for $5 week. They put on their "pitches" in the afternoons and evenings and slept in the wagon on the lot at night.

Customarily, True opened the show with a really marvelous performance of card tricks and magic. He pulled coins out of his ears and made huge tissue-paper flowers grow out of what seemed to be tiny seeds in his hand. Next, he preached on the virtues of his amazing medicinal mineral spirits, which sold for only $1 a bottle. Between pitches Wash played the banjo and sang Southern spirituals. The show usually lasted about two hours.

Edgar and True brainstormed how he could join the team. Edgar would need a dental chair. He imagined setting it upon the wagon, making his own "pitch" on dentistry and then pulling teeth in public demonstrations. Edgar also mentioned the idea of a friend who had suggested that he should refer to himself as the "painless dentist." True thought that was a splendid idea.

The plan suited Edgar, except for one minor detail. He didn't have a Washington dental license. True reassured him that would not be a problem. *"I was planning on taking the show southward into*

Oregon and California." True concluded, "I have looked up the laws in those states and all you will need is your diploma." Edgar took him at his word and did not give the license question another thought.

Edgar got his dental chair and learned his pitch. Things were going well. He was having the time of his life, doing his dental pitches, living in the back of a wagon and growing plump on Wash's Southern cooking. But once again, things were about to change.

One day while they were making a successful pitch in front of the Palace Hotel on Market Street in San Francisco, True suddenly decided that he wanted to go back to his ranch near Fort Whoop-Up in Alberta, Canada.

Although the long trip back was interesting, by the time they reached the ranch, their relationship had become somewhat strained. Eventually True and Edgar had to be separated by the 200-pound Wash during a fist fight. The disagreement was over what Edgar thought was a $2.50 swindle by True. The black eyes healed but the feeling never did, so in the summer of 1894 True and Parker parted ways.

While with True, Parker learned he could get some Alberta, Canada, land for nearly nothing. All one had to do was put up a barbed-wire fence around it and build a shack, and the Canadian government would let you have it for 10 cents an acre.

Edgar did just that around a four-mile area. He settled down in the ranch with several horses and a couple of dogs. But it didn't last. Out of the blue one day, another attack of "wanderlust" hit Edgar. He just walked off and left it all. He never knew what became of his ranch.

After spending several months wandering through the back-woods of central Canada, taking another bullet to the hat and almost being killed by Indians, Edgar decided it was time to return to St. John and try, once more, to be a regular office-practicing dentist.

However, before joining Edgar in New Brunswick, let's pause again and look at three important success principles he learned during this episode of his life.

The list of examples proving this principle is long. Soon after opening his first real "fixed" dental practice, Edgar realized that one dentist working alone is not productive. What if he would have had to deal with OSHA and HIPAA compliance, employee benefits packages, employee guidelines, insurance companies, federal, state and local government forms and regulations? The list goes on and will get longer with time. How much more unproductive time would he feel he was spending?

To stay in business today, every solo dental practitioner has to deal with all of this and more and, in the process, somehow treat patients. Edgar was right. One person by himself is not a productive model.

There are two ways a dentist can overcome this problem. Option one is: Invest the time and money to build systems and hire people to handle the unproductive tasks. Or have someone else set up a system. Option two can be done two ways: A dentist can hire a consultant who gets paid by the hour whether his or her plan works in the office; or like the Custom Dental model, the dentist can choose to partner with someone who has a proven system already in place. In this model, the only way Custom Dental succeeds is if the practice succeeds. The way I see it, Custom Dental has more skin in the game, therefore they are held more accountable.

Although William True was a questionable individual, Edgar learned a lot about self-promotion from him.

Several decades ago an evangelist-turned-entrepreneur shared an interesting story with me. On his Christian journey he had become a pastor of a small church in western Oklahoma. The church was so small it couldn't really pay him a salary. He and his family of four lived off the parsonage garden and what the members of the church would bring from time to time.

In his congregation there was a mentally slow 50-year-old single man who lived with his elderly parents. One Sunday, out of the kindness of his heart, the pastor invited the simpleton to have lunch with him and his family after church. During the course of the meal the pastor and his wife were having a discussion they thought exceeded the intellect of his two small children and the simpleton. The pastor was sharing his frustration about the general apathy of his congregation when the simpleton spoke up, *"Pastor, if everyone felt the same way you do, they would be pastors."*

That story and those words from the simpleton have been invaluable to me over the years.

Success leaves clues. They can be found in obvious places, such as with highly successful individuals. This is why I actively seek mentors and information from individuals like Dr. Tom Orent, Dan Kennedy, John Maxwell, Robert Echols and many others.

However, the clues can be found by listening and observing unsuspecting individuals such the pastor's dinner guest. I believe it is a Buddhist proverb that states, *"When the student is ready, the teacher will appear."* The secret to learning and applying this principle is staying ready.

Early in their relationship True taught Edgar this very important principle that would impact him for the rest of his life and, ultimately, influenced him to change his name.

As uncomfortable as self-promotion is for most folks, it is a common thread for everyone who has become extremely successful.

If you don't let the world know all your attributes, many will go unnoticed.

There is a whole book inside of me on self-promotion techniques. But for the purpose of this volume, let's just say, to be truly successful in dentistry, you must let people know why they should pick you to provide their care over all other choices. You are your product. You are what your patients buy. How are you packaging yourself?

Chapter Sixteen

ANOTHER ATTEMPT IN
NEW BRUNSWICK

*"I would rather entertain and hope that people learned something
than educate people and hope they were entertained."*

WALT DISNEY

B ACK to our story. Edgar had been away nearly two
years, and both his mother and father gave him a
heart-warming welcome back to St. Martin. His father's ship-chandlery business was nearly dead. Through his
ventures over the previous two years, Edgar had accumulated
some money, so he was pleased to help his parents with some
financial support.

After a few weeks he moved to St. Martin, where the showman
in him was emerging again. What was needed, as he saw it, was a
really big-time dentistry show—something to jar eastern Canada out
of its dental lethargy.

Edgar began looking for performers and, in no time, assembled
a large and strange troupe that was ready to go on the road.

Town and country folks flocked to stare at the war-whooping
braves, sword swallowers, bearded ladies, Irish tenors and belly
dancers. All of this took place while Dr. Parker, the painless dentist,
preached his tooth-care sermons from a gas-lighted podium.

In his hometown of St. Martin where Edgar had made 75 cents
for three months of dentistry a few years back, he was now bringing
in $250 a day with his traveling dental show.

After taking his Parker Comedian and Specialty Company on
a 60-day town circuit, filling streets and halls throughout Maine and

New Brunswick, Parker had a reflective, life-changing moment.

In the spring of 1895, at the tender age of 23, Edgar Randolph Rudolph Parker, D.D.S., took stock of his life. Although he was already a seasoned veteran of the road, Edgar was rapidly tiring of the country tooth pulling, visiting an endless string of villages and towns, performing open-air dental and medical stage shows and trying to keep one step ahead of the law.

Although he had achieved some monetary successes on the road and there had been plenty of day-to-day excitement, the overhead expenses of his medicine shows were excessive. By the time it was all said and done, his profits were not as good as he hoped.

Edgar was not the type to stay depressed too long. In his mind, the time had clearly come for him to abandon his traveling show and return to New York, where he had initially attended dental school.

While in New York, Edgar worked for another dentist. It brought in a meager income. Whenever he found himself tight financially, he fell back to his medicine shows and house-to-house dentistry to make ends meet. Eventually he found himself more back on the road and less in the traditional dentist office.

In May, 1896, Edgar went to Brooklyn to visit relatives. While there he ran into someone who would change his life forever. Frances Elizabeth Wolfe was a beautiful 19-year-old woman with big, expressive brown eyes that captured Edgar from the moment he saw her. Although Frances' father, Mr. Wolfe, was not impressed with Edgar as a suitable suitor for his daughter, Edgar and Frances had other ideas.

Before we find out what is in store for Edgar and Frances, let's disclose a few more success principles that Edgar had learned in this chapter of his life.

One Sunday in a Catholic service the assistant priest, fully cloaked in his robes, stood up at the front to the church and began to chant in a ceremonial tone and rhythm, *"I am the assistant priest of this church and I make only $500 a month."*

Not to be outdone in this opportunity to create sympathy from his congregation, just as soon as the assistant priest had completed

PRINCIPLE 40

There is power in reciprocity.

his melodious plea, the head priest immediately rose and chanted in the same tune, *"I am the priest of this church and I have invested uncountable hours to make only $700 a month."*

The dead silence of the congregation was suddenly broken when the giant organ pipes started and the organist's head appeared over the massive keyboard. He began to sing to his accompanying tune, *"I'm the organist in this church. I only show up for services and I make $4,000 a month. And there is 'No Business Like Show Business."*

How right that organist was. Basketball players, football stars and music entertainers all are some of the highest earners in our society. Why? Because people will pay for what they want. What do people want more than anything? To be entertained.

Savvy business owners, like Donald Trump, have that figured out. Very few dentists do.

You might ask, *"How can a dentist entertain?"* The answers are as varied as the number of smart dentists who ask it. I can give you a few examples, but I am afraid to say there is no "Easy Button" for it. You may have to actually think about this one. But, believe me, the time invested will be well worth it.

When I was in practice I bought small magic tricks. I would pull them off the shelf to amaze children and please moms.

I have a dental partner who is quite musically talented who frequently picks up a guitar and impresses his patients.

Whenever we have a promotional event we always try to bring in dancing dogs or inflatable play houses for kids or live bands for adults. Sometimes we even have our dental teams do skits. As crazy as it sounds, entertainment draws crowds, makes people laugh and, ultimately, lubricates future business transactions.

Very few dentists are aware of this powerful principle but those who are, do well.

Parker used this principle to ramp up his dental business from 75 cents in 90 days to $250 a day in the same community.

A few years back I got a call from a frantic dentist who wanted me to help him with his business. He had a six-office model, eight employed dentists and was generating around $7 million dollars gross, but he couldn't comfortably pull a paycheck.

PRINCIPLE 41

You only get one chance to make a good first impression.

I told him he could best use my $1,288 per hour consulting fee by gathering several statistics about his practice. Some of the statistics I needed included the breakdown of all his expenses.

I'm not sure why he had not tracked this on a regular basis, but after retrieving this information; his cash flow problems were obvious. His overhead was 104% of collections. This cash flow imbalance was only a symptom of many underlying problems. However, the point I want to make here is don't be fooled by the gross.

We use a monthly tracking system that calculates every expense item for each office and compares it to the group. This quickly allows us to make adjustments if necessary.

Edgar was wise, and you would be too, to not only track income but also expenses. A shrewd business mentor of mine said, *"God gave you two eyes, one to watch the income, the other to watch the expenses."*

Chapter Seventeen

PARKER WITH A NEW HAT, "HUSBAND"

"Efficiency is doing things right; effectiveness is doing the right things."

PETER DRUCKER

B Y August of 1896, Edgar believed that he had accumulated enough money to get married. He had heard
that Frances was at the town of Rosa Gap, New York,
visiting her married sister. He wrote her a letter telling her that
he wanted to marry her at once. Taking her affirmative answer
for granted, Edgar arrived on Saturday evening by train.

Edgar told her, *"Let's get married tomorrow!"*

"But tomorrow is Sunday," she protested.

"What of it?" Edgar replied. *"It will be all that easier to find a
preacher."*

So, on Sunday, August 2, 1896, they located a Parson Kerr at his
home shortly after noon. Edgar produced a $5 fee for the license and
wedding ring, and they were wed.

Edgar knew that he should take Frankie, a name he used for
Frances the rest of her life, back to Brooklyn as soon as possible to
make peace with her father, whom
he had met only briefly, and her
mother, whom he had never met.

PRINCIPLE 42

*Don't confuse busyness
with productivity.*

When they arrived in Brook-
lyn, the newlyweds stayed at Mrs.
Maine's house, where Edgar had lived part time while attending the
New York College of Dentistry.

Frankie left Brooklyn to visit her sister as Ms. Wolfe and returned as Mrs. Edgar Randolph Rudolph Parker. Frances' mother was shocked when Edgar introduced himself as her new son-in-law. Mr. Wolfe was so upset that he made Edgar show the marriage license before allowing him to enter their home.

Next, Edgar took his new bride to Vermont to introduce her to Jennie Parker, who was visiting relatives in the White Mountains.

After all the introductions and a week off work, Edgar was once again running out of money. It was time to get back to work. So they returned to New Brunswick and Edgar opened up a dental practice in a hotel in Moncton the following day.

The next day Edgar was once again turned into authorities by a local dentist and arrested for practicing dentistry without a license.

"I have a license," Edgar disputed.

The sheriff said, *"I don't know anything about that. All I know is that I have papers that clearly state that you're in violation of the law."*

Edgar told Frankie to go back home awhile and he would be back soon. Frankie didn't know the man who was with her husband was a sheriff. And Edgar didn't have the heart to tell her that her new husband was headed for the jail.

While Edgar was behind bars, he was charged $200 a day for the two days he had practiced in Moncton without a license.

Edgar discovered that the secretary of the local dental society, Dr. C.A. Murray, had heard of the notorious young renegade, Parker, setting up practice in his town. Dr. Murray knew that Edgar would not be privy to a regulation, a $2 registration fee, which had recently been passed to ensnare itinerant dentists. This was the society's big chance to nab Edgar.

Fortunately for Edgar, Cavor Chapman, the mayor of Moncton and a relative on his mother's side of the family, caught wind of what had happened to Edgar and promptly bailed him out. Edgar immediately paid the $2 fee, was re-instated as a practicing dentist and returned to his hotel office, only missing four hours of work.

Once again Edgar used the principle he learned in Vancouver in dealing with Dr. Jones: you can gather a big crowd by finding an enemy.

"Ladies and gentlemen," Edgar went on from his stage adjacent to Dr. Murray's office, *"if any of you here have received dental work by Dr. Murray that is not to your satisfaction, come to my office in the hotel and I will personally fix it for free."*

Edgar clearly won the public opinion and within a week of his constant attacked on Dr. Murray, that dentist went on extended vacation hoping things would eventually cool off.

Edgar's relatives heard word of his unprofessional conduct and wanted him to leave Moncton. Edgar replied, *"The average man seems to lie down in the face of trouble. I would have, but I was broke and on my own. I had no place to lie down. I had to fight back."*

In the fall of 1896, Edgar was making good money in dentistry but was still feeling a financial pinch. Because his father was facing the brunt of the ship-chandlery demise, Edgar was now supporting his parents, his siblings and his wife.

After Edgar had skimmed the cream off the top of the dental business in Moncton, it was time to move on. The next town the newlyweds lived in was Prince Edward Island, Canada, where Edgar opened hotel practice.

It didn't take him long to tire of the miserable Prince Edward Island weather. With a flip of a coin, he decided to go west to the warmer weather in Los Angeles.

Edgar gathered up enough money to take five people and two dogs to California on the Southern Pacific train. By this time his team consisted of a dental lab man, a fire eater, a cartoonist and two trained show dogs, all of which played an important part in Edgar's traveling dental show.

Things were not as lucrative in Los Angeles as Edgar had hoped. Economic times were tough there and the dental shows didn't bring in as many dollars as expected.

By January 1897, times had gotten so tough that Edgar's team disbanded and Edgar found himself working for Dr. Nathan T. Hale in an inside dental office in San Bernardino, California. Dr. Hale had another office in San Diego, so he allowed Edgar to run the one in San Bernardino. The dental office was in the front of the building, the master bedroom was in the middle room and Edgar's dental laboratory was in the back.

While in San Bernardino, Edgar ran across his old pharmacist friend who had helped him develop his wonder drug, hydrocaine. They started experimenting with the local anesthetic again. This time they added adrenalin and chloride to the concoction and found that it improved the drug's longevity of action. This was an improvement that is still used today.

In April, Frankie happily discovered that she was pregnant and immediately became homesick for Brooklyn. Edgar, realizing he couldn't send Frankie home without any money, turned the practice over to another dentist, rented a wagon and once again fell back on performing street dentistry and peddling patent medicines. Even after paying for their train tickets east, in six days he took in $1,286!

Wanting to show old man Wolfe that he had misjudged Edgar's capabilities to support his daughter, before leaving Los Angeles Edgar bought Frankie a diamond ring and some matching earrings.

On the long train trip home, Edgar had a lot of time to think. Finally he concluded, *"I'm a husband and soon-to-be father. I've got to learn how to deliver dentistry in a more conventional manner. The traveling dentistry lifestyle is not conducive to raising a family. Once and for all, I'm going to go straight."*

Edgar had $500 in cash by the time he and Frankie arrived in Brooklyn. The young Parkers stayed at the Wolfe's, where Dorothy Wolfe Parker was born on December 29, 1897.

Edgar's first job back in Brooklyn was working for Dr. George Gagnon, a dentist who owned one of the famous nationwide dental chains at the time, the New York Parlors.

Because of Edgar's heavy financial responsibilities, he needed to earn at least $180 a week to keep his head above water. Although he was making what was a good income working for Dr. Gagnon, he was unable to maintain the revenue he needed. Edgar found greener pastures in the Oyster Bay area of Long Island, New York, about 27 miles from downtown Brooklyn. At first Edgar made the commute, only coming home on weekends. However, by the summer of 1898 he was able to move Dorothy and Frankie to Sea Cliff, Long Island, to live with him.

PRINCIPLE 43

Advertising is not optional.

No matter how hard Edgar worked at his practice he was still making just enough to get by day-to-day. He felt his talent was being wasted in such a small community as Sea Cliff and thought if he could get located in a large community, things would be better.

One day while expressing his desires to a dental supply dealer, the man informed Edgar of a suitable location in downtown Brooklyn right across the street from the Long Island Railroad terminal. Although the building had been the home of two previous dentists who had failed miserably, Edgar's need to generate funds was pressing, so he rented the place for $75 a month, sight unseen.

PRINCIPLE 44

Don't waste your money on plain vanilla advertising.

By the time Edgar updated and converted the run-down office, he was once again left without a dime. This was the lowest point of his life. Here he was with a wife, a baby and no food in the cupboard.

His first day as a solo proprietary dentist was the longest in his life. He opened his doors at 10 A.M., but the first patient didn't show up until 9 P.M. that evening. This visit generated 75 cents to the fledgling practice. Edgar spent the first quarter in the gas meter so they could have heat; the remainder was spent for milk for the baby and some food for Frankie and himself.

Edgar rented his Brooklyn office from Colonel N.T. Sprague.

PRINCIPLE 45

If they aren't criticizing you, you must be doing something wrong or nothing at all.

Sprague employed William Beebe to take care of his properties and collect the rent. Beebe, a blue-eyed 6-footer tipping the scales at 300 pounds, avoided anything physical. He wore a mustache and combed his hair in a pompadour style. He continuously and nervously chomped on a long, black cigar. Beebe's main exercise was mental gymnastics. As it turns out he was one of the brightest people Edgar had ever met.

Beebe had been in the circus business for 45 of his 60 years. In fact, he had done almost everything in the P.T. Barnum Big Top including: feeding the animals; playing the slide trombone; and performing as a peanut vendor, advance man, talent scout, ticket seller and sideshow barker. In the circus, Beebe had learned the art and science of organization.

PRINCIPLE 46

Systems create the playing field for winning teams

At the time Edgar was the complete antithesis of organized. He had never had a bank account, made a deposit or written a check. And when it came to business, Frankie was just as naïve as her husband.

One day, when Edgar came to pay the rent, Beebe couldn't resist making an effort to straighten out this 26-year-old "kid." *"Doc,"* he said, *"why don't you help Uncle Sam out by writing a check, putting it in an envelope with a three-cent stamp, and sending it down here? Aren't you afraid that someone with some real money might show up at your office while you are coming over here to pay me?"*

Edgar, somewhat taken back, and missing the whole point of Beebe's comment, replied, *"It would take more time for me to get a money order and mail it to you than paying you personally in cash and getting a receipt."*

Beebe shook his head and said, *"That's a funny way of running a business."*

Edgar defensively retorted, *"Mr. Beebe, you need to realize I'm not a businessman, I'm a professional."*

"That's evident to me," concluded Beebe.

Edgar left the office not knowing whether he was being poked fun at or if Beebe was actually being sincere and helpful.

The next month when Beebe received the rent from Edgar, he took his sweet time filling out the receipt. When Edgar couldn't stand his poky pace any longer he said, *"Get a move on, Mr. Beebe. Time's a'wasting!"*

Beebe slowly and deliberately looked up and asked, *"If your time

PRINCIPLE 47
Technology can differentiate your practice.

is so valuable, why the hell don't you open a checking account and pay your rent the way everybody else does?"

Edgar tried to be indifferent to Beebe's question, trying to leave the impression he was far too occupied with professional matters to deal with such mundane issues as banking. However, truth be known, banking was a total mystery to Edgar.

During the first six months, few patients found their way to Edgar's second-floor dental office. As a result, he was sometimes late with the rent.

"Look, Parker," Beebe said after recognizing Edgar was struggling month to month, *"I don't mean to interfere with your life, but in my humble opinion you're just a dope! If you used circus methods, you'd soon be a millionaire!"*

Beebe went on to say, *"The other day I came up to your office. I intentionally coughed, kicked the paint nearly off your baseboard and made enough noise to raise the dead and you didn't even know I was there. I heard this 'tap, tap, tap.' I peeked around the corner and you were hitting someone's tooth with an instrument."*

PRINCIPLE 48
If you are going to butcher the pig, make sure to use the whole thing.

"I was pounding a gold foil," explained Edgar.

Beebe said, *"Maybe so. But you need a receptionist out in your parlor so that the ones with dough don't get away. When people go into a restaurant, they don't just stand there. They want to be noticed. To let folks cool their heels with no word of explanation is the kiss of death for any business."*

He was getting Edgar's attention.

Beebe continued as he picked up steam, *"Look, Doc, you have a wonderful future. I'm at the end of my trail, but if you want me to help you succeed beyond your wildest expectations, I'll do it. You need a manager. Why not give me a try?"*

"What kind of salary do you want?" asked Edgar.

Beebe thought a minute and said, *"Let's start off with $25 a month. You can pay me more when your financial situation improves."*

Edgar said he wanted to think it over and talk with Frankie before making a decision.

Beebe nodded as Edgar left.

PRINCIPLE 49
Many successes can be found and borrowed from outside industries.

After talking with Frankie, they both agreed they could afford Beebe and decided to hire him.

They both would have been shocked had they known what Beebe had in mind for Edgar's development. E.R Parker was about to be transformed and would soon launch his Parker's enterprises. But before we go there, let's reflect on a few principles Edgar added to his success tool kit.

The principle of reciprocity states, *"One is more likely to give you what you want if you first give them something they want."*

When Edgar addressed the crowd in Moncton, he was a bit upset and on the attack, but there was a method to his madness. He offered to correct Dr. Murray's work for FREE. After they got what they wanted, a free fix, Edgar was able to sell them more care.

At Custom Dental, we constantly give patients surprise gifts such as ice scrapers, lip balm, garden gloves, hot pad mitts and candles, to mention a few. Initially we gave these gifts after their care

PRINCIPLE 50
Make working for you more than a job.

when they were exiting the practice. Once we learned this principle, we reversed the gift giving and started passing them out before they went back for care. Our case acceptance went up. Do you think this might be the principle of reciprocity at work?

First impressions are lasting. A good first impression can set the stage for a long, meaningful relationship. A poor one may never be overcome.

Beebe's advice about getting a receptionist was a step in the right direction, but in my opinion he didn't go quite far enough.

PRINCIPLE 51

You can't get their money if they can't find you.

I would have added that Edgar needed a hospitable receptionist.

Most dentists aren't aware but this principle is violated in many offices. Typically our first impressions are made with new patients over the phone. How is phone being answered? Are you sure? How would you know? Most dentists are held hostage by their front desk and don't even know it. They are usually in the back tapping on teeth, as Beebe called it, and aren't hearing what is going on up front.

This is why Custom Dental monitors and grades all in-bound calls. Those team members needing help receive training and follow up. We also hire mystery shoppers who grade the entire dental experience. We are currently testing a surveillance system to assist us in consistently delivering a "World Class Dental Experience."

You might think I am a bit paranoid about delivering a "World Class Dental Experience." Well, you are right. I have monitored too many calls to know that being good on the phone is a difficult task and, if left to the discretion of a staff person, it can be inconsistent, at best, and down-right repelling, at worst.

First impressions can set the tone of your patient's attitude about you, your advice and your care. Make sure it is what you want it to be.

While Mary was preparing the traditional holiday ham, her husband, Bob, asked, *"Mary, I've always wondered why you cut two inches off each end of the ham before putting it in the cooker?"*

"I'm not really sure," Mary replied, *"I guess because my mom always did it that way."*

"I'm curious. Could you call her and find out why?" requested her husband.

Mary called her mom. *"Hi, Mom. Bob wanted to know why you cut two inches off each end of the ham before you put it in the cooker."*

Mary's mom replied, *"I'm not sure. Grandma always cut two inches off the ham before putting it in the cooker, so I've always done it that way myself."*

When Mary called Grandma and asked the same question, Grandma replied, *"Oh that's simple. The hams were always about 16 inches long and my cooker could only handle 12 inches."*

It took Beebe to open Edgar's eyes to the fact he didn't need to cut the end of the ham off any longer. His cooker could handle the 16-inch ham.

Because Edgar was always on the run, he had never used a bank account, made deposits or written checks. It was costing Edgar time and maybe patients using his old itinerant dentist systems in his new office model.

We are all victims of our own biases. That is why it is very beneficial to have a coach, mentor or, at least, an outside set of eyes to occasionally evaluate how we are doing things.

One of my dental coaches and a trusted mentor, Dr. Tom Orent constantly tests my biases. By doing so, he has opened the door to multiple opportunities.

The point is we can be so busy doing unnecessary or antiquated tasks that we can't grow, improve and become more productive.

Chapter Eighteen

EDGAR LEARNS ABOUT BEING A BUSINESS MAN

"Advertising is fundamentally persuasion and persuasion happens to be not a science, but an art."

WILLIAM BERNBACH

EDGAR quickly got back with Beebe. *"Mr. Beebe, you're the man. You call the shots."*

Beebe said, *"Well for starters, drop the mister, and call me 'Bill.' I need to know your story, your life as a dentist and what you have done to promote yourself since graduating from dental school."*

For the next hour or so, Edgar shared every episode of his life with Beebe. Beebe knew he had found a suitable student to whom to impart his knowledge. Edgar had already been doing many things right; however he had no organization, systemization or follow up.

Beebe said, *"At this point, Doc, we need to change and enlarge your attitudes about advertising."*

PRINCIPLE 51

You can't get their money if they can't find you.

Beebe pulled a tattered copy of *The Autobiography of P.T. Barnum* from his desk and said, *"Let's see what an expert on the subject has to say about it."*

Beebe carefully opened the book to page 156 and said, *"Look at these passages, especially the ones I have underlined."*

Edgar read the following words:

Whatever your occupation or calling may be, if it needs support from the public, advertise it thoroughly and efficiently, in some shape or

other, that will arrest public attention...There may possibly be occupa-
tions that do not require advertising, but I cannot well conceive what
they are...Some say 'they cannot afford to advertise;' they mistake—
they cannot afford not to advertise...As a businessman, undoubtedly,
my prime object has been to put money in my purse...

Barnum reiterated that he could say successful advertising was the reason he succeeded beyond his expectations, and he was satisfied.

Edgar took in all of Beebe's advertising advice.

"Doc, whatever you do," Beebe advised, *"if you spend money for a sign or for advertising, do not, under any circumstances, make it ordinary. Make it so that whoever sees it will stop, look and listen. Being nice has its limitations. There are enough people already working that side of the street."*

Beebe added, *"Do nothing you can hire someone else to do, as long as you can make at least a 10% profit."*

In his discussions with Beebe, Edgar attempted to justify the premise that professionals don't really need to advertise.

Beebe countered with, *"But suppose, Doc, that you continue doing nothing undignified and the patients continue to stay away, what then? Are you going to let your family starve?"*

Edgar tried to explain that the ethical way for a professional to advertise would be to join the right clubs, be seen in the right places and meet the right people.

After Edgar presented his case, Beebe remarked, *"Doc, if that's true, why aren't you out there right now mingling and making those social contacts?"*

Edgar sheepishly replied, *"Well, Bill, moving about in such circles costs a lot of money and takes too much time. I don't have enough of either."*

Gradually Beebe was convincing Edgar of the fact that if a dentist advertised, it didn't necessarily mean he was a "quack" or a poor dentist. Beebe illustrated the point by using Barnum, who was an example of a highly moral, upright individual who had done a great deal of good for society but was misunderstood and upbraided by society for not following what they considered the rules.

He commented about Barnum's criticism, *"Doc, Barnum had a healthy attitude about others' criticism and turned it around or deflected it. There is a price for being ahead of your time, but there is a worse price staying in the pack."*

Edgar knew Bill was 110% right and said, *"All right, Bill, I surrender. I just needed to fully convince myself that this is the right course for me and my family. You are my manager, so tell me what to do."*

Edgar had decided to buy back into **Principle 3: Differentiate or Die.**

At that moment, Brooklyn's regular dental ranks were decreased by one. Edgar was about to enter on a program that would keep organized dentistry in intermittent turmoil for the next 50 years. Edgar might later have moments of reservation, but essentially he would not look back. This was it!

Beebe went on, *"Good! Excellent decision. We're going to go about this process in an orderly and systematic way. The circus has survived and prospered over the years because hundreds of men, from the top bosses down to the lowliest roustabouts, each had his particular job to do and did it. Systems, my boy! That's what is going to make you rich."*

"For advertising purposes," Beebe added, *"you'll need to drop the 'E.R. Parker' name and revert back to the old moniker that you so successfully used in Canada, 'Painless Parker.' There are already four other Dr. Parkers practicing dentistry in Brooklyn. We need to help people go to the 'right' one. Drop the 'E.R.', your name is now 'Painless Parker.' You got that? I'm never calling you Edgar again."*

Beebe went on to show what signage he had in store for Painless Parker's office. All were emphatic, bold, big and could be seen from a mile away.

Beebe then advised Painless that he would once again need to hit the streets with his outdoor dental demonstrations until Parker's name was better known.

Each evening for several weeks, Painless and Beebe rented an open carriage and drove it to the busiest corners in Brooklyn, the Bronx and Coney Island. At the appointed time, Beebe would stand in the carriage and play his slide trombone to attract a crowd. Then Beebe would announce, "Ladies and gentlemen! Boys and girls! It is my pleasure to introduce you to Dr. Painless Parker, the noted pioneer in painless dentistry. For your benefit and enlightenment, Dr. Parker will deliver his celebrated and world-famous educational lecture on dental hygiene. Pay close attention, please, this is a vital subject!"

Painless would then stand and give his standardized and well-rehearsed dental sermon. After Painless had finished, Beebe would briefly speak about the doctor's crusade to bring down the cost of dentistry to within the reach of the masses. Parker would also guarantee he was truly painless. The crowd was urged to waste no time showing up at his second-floor office in Brooklyn, with very specific instructions on how to get there.

The night talks and signs immediately increased the number of patients showing up at Painless' office.

One day, Beebe took Painless aside and showed him a piece of paper. He said, *"Doc, remember, I am here to teach you some basic success principles. Look at this list."*

Painless read the following:

To be successful

1. *Learn how to sell.*
2. *Learn how to attract attention to you and your business.*
3. *Learn how to borrow working capital.*
4. *Learn that it isn't you know, but by you are known.*

Thereafter, Painless would refer to this list, calling it his "blueprint for life." Not bad advice for anyone.

Beebe continued to make good on his promise of getting Painless attention. He hired banjo players, acrobats and magicians for his outside dental shows. He hired tight-rope walkers to walk a rope in pink tights outside Edgar's office window to draw attention to the new signage. He even arranged a Sunday afternoon parade with the featured guest being Parker, who was royally dressed complete with top hat. There was also a bugler who announced Painless to the observers.

Eventually Painless was confronted with far more patients than he could handle. Beebe informed him he would have to install modern business methods to keep up with the increased demand.

Within a matter of weeks, Painless hired a receptionist and an office assistant and the office expanded to take over the entire second floor of the building. A few months later, the third floor was added, and now he began to hire other dentists, lab men and office help. While Painless supervised the professional staff, Beebe systematized the operations by which a steady stream of patients kept flowing through the business.

Beebe's special pride was the installation of a mechanized Lamson Cash Carrier System, which served to move money efficiently around the two floors. But more importantly, it brought in hundreds of Brooklynites who came to satisfy their curiosity about how this modern machine worked, to then eventually become patients.

In those days, telephones were far less common. Beebe, in his campaign to convince the public that the Parker office was the last word in modern dentistry, had wall phones installed beside every third dental chair. It worked. In their minds, Painless Parker was decidedly a new-world experience.

Beebe had taken an individual who was on the brink of disaster, breathed life into him and made him the talk of the town. Painless, like a dry sponge, was soaking up all of Beebe's circus experience.

With the combination of Beebe's direction and Parker's energy, the two-floor Painless Parker dental office grew beyond the capacity of one office. Eventually they had to find other locations.

Painless Parker, who had trouble paying a $27.50 office lease less than two years earlier, was now the owner and operator of 17 offices producing over $1M in the New York area.

Life was good for the Parker family. Painless bought a beautiful beach-front estate outside of Brooklyn between Bath Beach and Coney Island. He raised high-bred horses and hired a cook and a chauffeur. Beebe was right. The circus advertising and systems had made Painless rich.

By this time, Painless was so much involved with his public appearances and with the administration of his 17 offices that he had given up the actual practice of dentistry. However, if an occasion arose for some worthwhile publicity, Parker could be counted on coming out of retirement.

One such occasion was to pull an ulcerated tooth from Leo, King of the Beasts, in the center ring of the circus. Although Painless initially baulked at the idea, Beebe convinced him to go forward with it. As usual, Beebe's idea was a hit. Parker's name was a topic of conversation at every home and place of business for weeks. It worked so well that in later years at a Pacific coast circus, Painless pulled a hippopotamus tooth.

Although Painless offered wages far higher than the average dentist could earn in private practice, it was a continual challenge to find enough qualified persons to handle his steadily increasing number of new patients. As it were, most new dental graduates wanted an independent practice. Most could not afford the investment, so they would work for Painless until they had enough money, then leave to start their own practice.

The other challenge Parker had was that most dentists felt there was something wrong about working for an advertising dentist. Even if they could overcome the stigma, sometimes their families couldn't.

Parker finally arrived at a very innovative method to obtain qualified dentists who would be willing to stay. Painless soon realized that dentists who were down-and-out drunks could be a rich source of employees. In fact, some of his most productive operators were peoples who had once had lucrative practices of their own but had drunk themselves out of business. Parker would rehabilitate them by sending them to a sanatorium to dry out and steady up. He gave them new clothes, helped them with their debts and gave them hope and a job again. He enjoyed the process and the challenge of salvaging human beings. As he put it, *"Sometimes it's necessary to turn a man around and face him in a better direction. It's like putting a square peg into a square hole even if you have to make the hole yourself."*

Painless believed that the nervous tension and time pressures generated by dentistry were responsible for driving some to use alcohol or drugs.

In time, the word got out that Painless Parker was offering jobs to anyone who could rehabilitate himself. As a result, alcoholic dentists from all over the East Coast began to locate Painless.

Parker claimed that he had worked with so many alcoholics that he could determine which ones would be a good risk after talking with an applicant for just a few minutes.

Although some rehabilitated dentists left him after a year or two to successfully re-establish themselves in private practice, Painless did not bear any hard feelings towards them. He felt good that he could help these "hopeless wrecks" get their lives back together. However, many of his rehabilitated dentists remained and were put in charge of branch offices. They eventually became important cogs in what became the "E.R. Parker Systems."

PRINCIPLE 52

A successful model can be duplicated.

Unfortunately late in 1902, Beebe suffered a massive stroke, and died within three days. Although Painless didn't realize it at the time, this marked the beginning of the end for his Brooklyn life episode.

Eventually Parker would establish the Painless Parker Training Center where he would train dentists and staff members the Painless Parker way of doing dentistry. He also started a profit-sharing plan. These additions provided employment glue to his company.

Painless also discovered that dentists and employees had abilities for some things and weaknesses for others. He started segregating the work based on their strengths. He had some dentists who were good at pulling teeth and others who were skilled at making dentures. A patient would ultimately be routed to the appropriate person to provide the service they did best. *(Parker used what he had learned at sea and Principle 21.)*

Parker was very particular were he established his new offices. They had to be in a highly visible area and comfortable for his patients to visit.

Before we continue with Parker's ascension, let's glean a few more practice success principles.

Researchers have determined that we are bombarded daily by over 3,000 advertising messages. If you expect to be found, you must use some form of advertising. If you follow Beebe and many other successful business builders, you will use several different marketing messages packaged in multiple media formats.

At Custom Dental we may use as many as 20 marketing sources at one time. Once I was asked by a seminar attendee, "Do you know of a marketing campaign that can bring in 100 new patients?"

PRINCIPLE 53

No one has ever snuck up on success.

My answer was, *"No. But I do know of a 100 marketing campaigns that can bring in one."*

What Beebe told Painless is even more important today, *"Doc, whatever you do, if you spend money for a sign or for advertising, do not, under any circumstances, make it ordinary. Make it so that whoever sees it will stop, look and listen. Being nice has its limitations. And there are enough people already working that side of the street."*

As I stated earlier, if your patients are being hit with over 3,000 advertising messages a day, you have to be very creative in getting their attention.

There are stacks of books written on this topic, and whether you do your own marketing or have a "Beebe" do it for you, I suggest you familiarize yourself with those resources. How can you evaluate this very important part of your business, if you know nothing about it?

As long as Edgar was barely surviving, practicing dentistry like all the others, no one was criticizing him. As soon as he stepped out of the box his peers and even his family, began to criticize him. Some of his peers even used dental boards to attack him.

When I first started advertising I had many business owners in town, some of the other dentists and even my own employees criticize my tactics.

In 2001 when I started to look for financing for what was to become Custom Dental, I had to go to six different banks. After explaining my plan, most the bankers looked at me like I had left my morning breakfast on my chin.

I was turned into the dental board for false advertising by a jealous dentist at one of my practice locations. We had to verify every testimony displayed in all our written and online advertising. I was even criticized for a statement I made in one of my books, *The Official Hand Guide for Picking Your Dentist,* when I said *"50% of all dentists graduate in the bottom half of their class."* Really, what is wrong with that?

There is no other way to plate this. Criticism is always the side dish served with success.

As you can tell by this part of Parker's story, systems became the backbone for everything they did in the Painless Parker enterprise. At first, Painless became a systems student. Eventually he became the teacher.

When I left for Glendale, California, in 1987 for my first life-changing seminar, it was not a dental training course. It was a business course. After five full days of studying systems and how I could implement them into my practice, I was on my way.

As the Founder and Chairman of Custom Dental, my main jobs are developing, training, evaluating and enforcing systems. We are continually tweaking operational manuals, training programs and monitoring systems.

Many dentists try to operate a practice with vague or even non-existent systems and wonder why they are living in chaos with little to show for their efforts. Developing operating systems demands working as hard on your practice as you work in it.

Beebe taught Painless how to re-invest back into his practice by buying technology.

Many of my dental school classmates have not made any technology changes in their offices since Jimmy Carter took office. When I see them at meetings, they say things like, *"Me and computers don't mix."* Or even more pathetic, *"I would go digital, but I can't justify the investment at my age."* These guys have fallen asleep at the technology wheel and will find themselves awakened in the practice-shrinking ditch.

At Custom Dental we are constantly investigating technology. If we find something we think can help our patient experience or increase our efficiency, we will test it at one location. If we find it is beneficial, we roll it out to the rest. A typical new patient comment as they observe all of our new technology is, "I've never been in a dental office like this."

Buying the right technology is not easy. You want to be on the cutting edge, not the bleeding edge. If not done properly, a dentist can end up with a closet full of gadgets that he has exchanged for his retirement. However you don't want to try convincing your patients that 1980 dental technology is as good as it gets.

When I was growing up, we lived next to a neighbor who raised and butchered one hog a year. It was usually a family ceremony. The hog was shot and strung up in a tree, then the process would start. By the end of the day, there was absolutely nothing left of that hog, not even his ears.

Beebe was an expert at "butchering the hog." The Lamson Cash Carrier System and the wall phones were great examples of his promotional leverage. He not only improved the office efficiency with technology he also added new patients to the practice by promoting it.

Beebe used many of the P.T. Barnum techniques and systems to build the Parker Empire, everything from the way they advertised and promoted the practice to how they systematized the operations.

I have borrowed many ideas from outside industries to build Custom Dental: the organizational board, employee compensation programs and marketing campaigns, to mention a few. I found these ideas by attending meetings and reading materials from businesses outside dentistry.

One of the biggest mistakes most dentists make is limiting their education. They go to dental seminars, read dental publications and end up implementing programs and systems just like the rest of their peers. This incestuous habit makes it very difficult, if not impossible, to differentiate their practices from the rest.

Parker found himself in the people-building business. As messy as that business is, it is the most rewarding. When you have systems in place so your team can be exposed to personal development programs, three great things happen. First, it repels those who are not interested in getting better. Next, those who buy into the growth culture become better. When they become better the team gets stronger. Last, when you empower a team member to become better, the principle of reciprocity kicks in and they become a loyal advocate of you and your practice.

One evening I was at a cocktail party discussing this principle with someone who was responsible for a team in the oil and gas industry. He said, "You are absolutely right. I constantly talk with my team about how they need to get better to face the stress of the day."

However, when I inquired, *"So what programs do you have in place to help them grow?"* he took a big gulp of his cocktail and wandered off looking for a refill.

At Custom Dental, we have implemented monthly leadership, character development, production, administrative and Doc's mastermind meetings as well as quarterly personal development seminars. We also conduct an annual conference focusing on both professional and personal development. Becoming a better person at work and at home has become part of our culture. As I look back, we continually reap the three benefits I have mentioned above.

Most dentists go to work, fix teeth and go home. Consequently, they find themselves surrounded by a bunch of clock punchers and they wonder why. As the controversial motivational speaker, Larry Winget, puts it, *"If your business sucks, it is because you suck."* I will say, *"If your dental team sucks, it is because you suck as the team leader."* The messy part about building people is that to be successful at it, you must first work on yourself, and then continue that process forever.

Once Parker caught Beebe's vision he became very particular where he placed his practices. He wanted highly visible locations.

We track our new patient source like a coon dog on a hunt and we constantly find a large percentage of them come from our outside signage. We build our offices in the main flow of the community and place the largest allowable signs in front of them. We sometimes spend what most dentists would consider a premium amount for our location, but we consistently find it pays.
During the construction of one of our offices I got a call from a concerned dentist-partner, *"We just got a nasty letter from someone in the neighborhood about how ugly and unprofessional our sign is. Do you think we need to change it?"*

I chuckled and said, *"I wouldn't change that sign if the little whinny complainer paid for it himself."*

After my partner got 50 new patients from the sign the first month he opened his doors, he became a believer in ugly, unprofessional signs.

While considering locations for new Custom Dental offices, we will survey the prospective community for several things. One of our prime considerations is the location of all the rest of the dentists in that community. It amazes me where some dentists locate their offices. Sure, a better location may be more expensive but consider this, if it costs $200,000 more, that breaks down to about $2,000 a month more overhead, one root canal and a crown. We have found that a visible location with good signage will bring in more than one toothache a month.

Chapter Nineteen

PARKER TAKES A BREAK?

"Be daring, be different, be impractical, be anything that will assert integrity of purpose and imaginative vision against the play-it-safers, the creatures of the commonplace, the slaves of the ordinary."

CECIL BEATON

IN 1906, at the age of 34, Parker had come to the realization that he was pooped. His mental health was taking a beating, and he wasn't sure he could continue.

Parker later wrote, *"After nine years of the hardest kind of work, I found myself with a half a million dollars in the bank and on the brink of having a second nervous breakdown."*

He decided he wanted to retire and become a gentlemen farmer and racehorse breeder in California. Another benefit in moving to California would be putting the width of the entire continent between himself and all of his relatives, most of whom he was on bad terms with.

His brother Hal, who had become a dentist, and his father were trading on the Parker name and operating competing "ethical" dental offices. Members of both families resented Painless' flamboyant, shoot-from-the-hip style, staged theatrics and blatant advertising. They thought Edgar was working to undermine the family's good social standing.

After selling Frankie on the move, Painless started to sell his business and personal holdings, although he didn't totally divest himself from some of his business properties for another 15 years.

In October of 1906, Parker had retired. He packed up his belongings, seven expensive racehorses and a newly purchased motor car and shipped them by rail in two cattle cars to Los Angeles, California, with his family following close behind.

When Painless left New York he told his relatives, *"I am going to relax for keeps!"* He probably meant it, at least for awhile. But the energy of the young and growing California eventually stirred his blood to a boil, forcing him back into action.

From the start, Painless couldn't stop himself from quietly studying the local dental situation in Los Angeles. In his customary and neat penmanship he would record a log of the dental advertisements that appeared in the *Los Angeles Times*. He was surprised to find eight advertising dentists within a six-block radius in downtown Los Angeles.

In his new life Parker had ample time to consider his situation. He was 34, a married professional man with plenty of money, a very attractive wife and three lovely daughters. Wasn't that enough out of life? What was he trying to prove anyway? As hard as he tried to convince himself he should be happy, he couldn't quite get there.

One day, while strolling with Frankie through his orange groves, she said to him, *"Dear, I know you are not happy. You pace around here like a caged cat. You need some way to let out that pent-up energy. What are you going to do about it?"*

Of course, she was not suggesting that he start another "unethical" dental practice. She proposed that perhaps he could invest in a respectable, low-key business venture. After all, he had enough money to do so.

Painless poured over newspaper advertisements and considered buying another orange grove. A few hours before making the final decision, he noted that there was a one-story building occupied in part by a small, emaciated, pathetic-looking, non-advertising dentist named J.F. Fram.

Fram worked in a shabby, one-room parlor, resembling the room that Painless had occupied during his worst moments in Brooklyn.

It was clear to Parker that, if ever there were an individual who needed to be "rescued" it was Dr. Fram. He thought, *"This guy is going to starve to death. I can turn this guy around and in the process do what I did in New York!"*

That night after opening a bank account with $500 for the new venture with Fram, there was a terrific struggle within Painless between the "showman" and the "respectable, ethical man." The respectable man whispered, *"It's insanity for you to consider starting a third career at the age of 34. Are you crazy? How can you do this to Frankie again? How will she be able to handle the stress of the inevitable criticism of being married to such a renegade? You know you will be hounded by dentists and dental boards."*

Painless awoke the next day certain about who won the imaginary argument that night. Immediately, Painless apologetically announced to Frankie, *"I have this itch that I simply must scratch."*

He put on his bullet-ridden top hat, his tails, ascot tie and spats and strutted out the door with 12 carats of diamonds on his hands. What a sight!

He drove to Dr. Fram's office and told him, *"Get your forceps limbered up. You're gonna need 'em. I'm gonna go out on the streets and dig up some worms!"* He acquired a loud electric horn, a set of Swiss bells and a small portable organ.

That morning, Painless drove his new red Peerless automobile, which had a big round sign on the side with Parker's name, to downtown Los Angeles and parked in the busiest intersection he could. He short-circuited the Peerless so it would backfire, set off a string of firecrackers next to the car, cranked up the electric horn and rang the bells

In a matter of minutes, Painless was standing up in his auto, and he began his famous lecture on the terrors of tooth neglect. Also in a matter of minutes, a patient was sitting in the Peerless rumble seat about to become the first person to experience a public tooth-pulling demonstration on Painless' comeback.

That afternoon and the rest of the week, patients flocked to Dr. Fram's office. By mid-week Dr. Fram was mentally and physically exhausted. Painless soon rented more rooms in the building, brought in rocking chairs and soap boxes in order to have more make-shift dental chairs. In a short time Painless hired more dentists on a commission basis and began to run advertisements in the local newspapers.

Within two months, four Painless Parker dental offices had opened in Los Angeles and their combined receipts were averaging

$1,000 a day, which in today's money would be equivalent to about $75,000. Frankie was totally disgusted and disappointed and refused to talk to him. The quiet Dr. Fram silently disappeared one day, never to show his face again. Painless remarked when he found out, *"He must have been terrified of prosperity."*

Painless continued at a neck-break pace. He eventually hired a film maker to make his films on dental education, hired a sign painter and cartoonist, contracted a pilot and airplane to drop flyers out in the streets and even bought a circus, all to promote the Painless Parker dental offices.

As expected, Parker was attacked by peers and dental regulators. Painless' patients were paid to file lawsuits against him.

Painless eventually took and passed several Pacific Coast state dental board exams, as he expanded his operation into neighboring states. He ultimately built 28 Painless Parker offices located in California, Oregon, Washington and British Columbia. Some of these offices had as many as 17 working dentists.

In the 1914 – 15 session of the California legislature, a bill was introduced that would forbid anyone to practice dentistry under any name other than their official name.

Parker was alarmed. He remembered a similar law being passed in 1905, which was one of the reasons he left New York. There was absolutely no question that Painless was becoming "target number one" in another state.

As soon as the bill was passed Parker immediately started a process to officially change his name to Painless. Although his first attempt was denied in the courts of Marin County, he placed a new petition in the Superior Court of the State of California and on September 15, 1915, Edgar Randolph Rudolph Parker officially became Painless Parker. Eventually Painless filed incorporation papers with California's secretary of state to form the "Painless Parker, Dentist" corporation. Painless had won the battle.

Parker eventually opened the Parker Institution of Dental Economics to recruit and train dentists, dental assistants and lab technicians into the E.R. Parker Systems of doing dentistry. The institute was opened and provided services to the public at cost. After training, most of the dentists, 95% of the assistants and two-thirds of the technicians remained in the Parker System.

In 1921, Painless hired Seth C. Maker, D.D.S., a former state dental board president, as his publicity man. Maker not only added to Parker's credibility he was also responsible for launching Painless' first radio show. The daily program aired at noon and was heard by an estimated audience of 3,000 in a 400-mile radius around Long Beach, California. His radio program eventually became affiliated with the National Broadcasting Company, and Painless could be heard weekly on Friday night at 9:45 P.M. on the NBC station KPO.

In January of 1924, Painless launched the first issue of "Occlusion," a 24-page company publication that presented the details of the E.R. Parker System dental offices. It was a publication that promoted his system, principles and core values and all the benefits of being in the Parker system.

Parker's momentum carried over into the realm of dental supplies as well. He developed Painless Parker mouthwash and toothpaste and many other dental hygiene products.

Early in 1924, Parker also established a profit-sharing plan for all the participating dental associates. In June of that year, he established a group insurance plan in which E.R. Parker Systems paid a portion of the premiums.

The next 28 years were not easy for Painless. He continued to aggressively expand his model. Although he was a man ahead of his time, his peers did not appreciate his approach. Parker was frequently the target of dental boards, lawyers and jealous dentists. Throughout his lifetime he spent hundreds of thousands of dollars defending his methods of advertising.

Ned, Parker's only son, was a constant disappointment to him. Although Ned followed his father's footsteps into dentistry, he was constantly plagued with breakdowns, divorces and alcoholism. Once he became a licensed dentist, he would have nothing to do with Painless or his dental empire.

His wife, Frankie, died of complications of a stroke on August 16, 1943, just two weeks after she and Painless celebrated their 47th wedding anniversary.

Against all obstacles, including his own health issues, Painless continued to preach, through advertising, his message of educating the public about dental care. He died on November 8, 1952, at the age of 80.

On September 22, just 47 days before his death, and despite the protest of Miss Lederer, his personal secretary, Parker came out of his sick bed with a burst of energy and worked from 9:30 A.M. until 5:00 P.M. "selling and extracting teeth" because one of his recovering alcoholic dentists had fallen off the wagon.

Although Parker's life is an example for anyone who wants to succeed in any business, his death was an example of what happens when you refuse to prepare for a transition. Maybe his rocky relationship with Ned made him hesitate. Maybe Edgar thought some day they would work things out and he could trust his son with the Parker Empire, but this never happened. As a matter of fact within the first year after Parker's death, a few well-meaning people in the E.R. Parker organization reached out to Ned to see if he would take over the Parker helm.

We don't know what Ned's response was, but it was generally known and accepted in the Parker family that he was not interested in taking over his father's reins.

By mid-1954, individual state-board decrees to remove the Painless Parker signage effectively killed the E.R. Parker Systems as a separate operating entity in the Pacific Northwest.

For whatever reason, Painless had not prearranged for an orderly succession of leadership or for the resolution of financial matters after his death.

It eventually took 12 years to settle Frankie's estate and 7 years to take care of his. In the end after the lawyers and creditors were taken care of there was hardly any money left to distribute to the heirs.

Shortly before Parker died, his daughter, Jane, told him *"Dad, when you die, the Parker System will die also. It will be like a group of Arabs on the desert who, one day, fold up their tents and silently disappear."*

That is exactly what came to pass.

There are many principles to be learned in Painless' life and also in his death.

Although Parker was encouraged by many to stop or consider another career, his very core principles would not let him. The moment he saw poor Dr. Fram struggling to make a living it ignited a response that even Painless, himself, could not stop. Within 24 hours of making the decision to jump back into dentistry, he was back out on the street doing what had worked in New York.

The first 10 years of my professional career resembled Moses wandering in the desert. The next 10 years I went from the bottom of the heap to the top. In 2001, I had a close friend and colleague retiring from his career as a dentist in the Indian Health Service approach me about associating with me in my practice. I had attempted and failed miserably at adding associates to my practice in the past, so I was very hesitant in risking our friendship on a busted associate agreement.

Instead I offered to partner with him in a practice in a community 30 miles north of Guthrie, Oklahoma. I would provide the capital, systems and knowhow and he would provide the dental care. Within a short time the new practice flourished. My son Nathan, who graduated from dental school, partnered with me and opened our third location in 2007. A few of his classmates caught word about what we were doing, and the rest is history. Currently I am partnering in 10 locations, with several applicants for future sites in progress.

Although our expansion process becomes smoother with each practice launch, the core values and operational systems are nothing more than a duplication of my original successful practice.

What are you doing that is working? Can you systematize it so someone else can duplicate your success? If so, the final question is, "What size do you want your check?" With diligent effort, it can be whatever you want it to be. Parker did it. I did it. You can do it.

When Painless finally gave into his calling, his next move was an all-out attack. He didn't spend time rearranging Dr. Fram's office or making sure his books were in order. Parker immediately hit the street with both barrels firing to the point of literally hauling patients to the office.

I believe I have launched more operator-owned solo practices than any other dentist in the world. We have carefully designed a multifaceted opening campaign that guarantees patients piling in the doors on the first day. In some markets we have had as many as 110 new patients on the appointment book before we opened for business.

I am amazed when I see a dentist opening a new practice like a youngster would approach opening a roadside lemonade stand. They make the lemonade, throw out a cardboard sign saying "Lemonade for Sale $1" and expect a crowd to show up.

Gary Halbert, a marketing legend, puts it this way, *"The money doesn't come from your service or product. It's in the selling of your service or product."*

The next time you get excited at a dental seminar about a new dental technique or service and before you plop down your good money on the gizmo that will make it possible, find yourself a quiet corner and ask these questions, *"How can I create the demand?"* and *"How can I sell it?"* Answering those two questions first, will save and make you a pile of money.

John Maxwell, a well-known international leadership guru says, *"Nothing of any magnitude has ever been accomplished by one. It takes a team."* The only way to recruit, motivate and maintain a team is with a vision big enough to be magnetic.

PRINCIPLE 54

Vision separates the "haves" from the "have nots."

As you can tell by Parker's history, Painless always had a team. From inspiring his sister, Bessie, with visions of their own chicken business to convincing his friend, Jack, to join him on a venture to the west, Painless always spun the dream of a better tomorrow. There are multiple examples in Parker's life where he utilized this principle, but I have chosen to highlight a few in his later years.

In a world where Painless felt that organized dentistry was depriving the multitudes of dental services, he used many tools to share his vision. He shared this vision with those in the Parker system through his intercompany publication "Occlusion" and many other speeches and publications.

He stood behind that vision by offering at-cost dental care to patients at his E.R. Parker Systems training center.

Another technique he used to get vision buy-in was by offering profit sharing to the Painless Parker dental associates. When the team feels they have some ownership in the vision they will fight for it.

The core value that pulled my practice out of the ditch and set it on a historical path was a deep understanding of who we were and who we served. Today we still believe that Custom Dental is on a mission of delivering "World Class Dental Experiences" by building the people inside our walls.

Personal growth of every individual from the partnering dentists to the part-time employees is a constant mission at Custom Dental. We have almost weekly meetings focusing on leadership skills, self improvement programs and character development. We host quarterly seminars and annual conferences where we bring in guest experts from all over the country to build our teams. Custom Dental even has its own internet resource center where team members can access self development and leadership resources.

Many of my peers think I am crazy, but the money we invest in these types of programs has a tremendous ROI. Our growth culture does two very important things: It attracts team members who want more than a paycheck, and it repels those who don't.

By constantly reminding about and clarifying the vision of delivering "World Class Dental Experiences" with highly-skilled, personally-mature individuals, Custom Dental is making a difference in the communities we serve and the lives of those who buy into it.

The first 10 years of my practice, my vision was getting out of bed and dragging my butt into a depressing office to put up with disappointed patients and disgruntled staff one more day. Not a very big vision, and it attracted no one. What is your vision?

As I became fascinated with this man named Edgar Randolph Rudolph Parker, "Painless Parker," I was shocked at how few people had ever heard of him.

Painless was a dental renegade. He was one of the first dentists to use local anesthetic. His out-of-the box approach to the profession was very instrumental in the formation of dental boards across the country. Painless owned the Painless Parker Circus. He had a long-standing media series, **Painless Parker Outlaw, His Confessions,** in many publications like the **San Francisco Bulletin,** which was later published as a 32-page pamphlet. In 1948, Hollywood cast Bob Hope as Painless Parker and Jane Russell as Calamity Jane in "The Paleface," a 91-minute Technicolor farce inspired by the incidents in Painless' early life.

PRINCIPLE 55

The difference between success and significance is legacy.

To say that Parker had made an impact on dentistry in his lifetime would be an understatement. Yet when I asked the people from his home town; dental graduates from his dental alumni, Temple University; or dental peers no one seems to know who he was.

Maybe it was the lifelong conflict with his son, the early death of his wife or just his preoccupation with what was happening in the moment, but Painless failed miserably at transmitting his tremendous efforts into the future.

After the unexpected loss of a son in 1987, I realized that there were no promises for tomorrow. I believe in life's cycle of learn, earn and then return. As I reflect back on the six decades of my life, it is very apparent that it is now my time to return.

I work hard every day to protect and project the Custom Dental culture into the future in hopes that it will affect lives long after I am gone.

Although Painless missed his opportunity, I hope you will glean a few principles from my attempt to pass on the "Painless Parkers Principles for Practice Success" that will make a difference in your life. And if you do, please keep the legacy alive. Pass it on.

Chapter Twenty

PAINLESS PARKER'S PRINCIPLES FOR PRACTICE SUCCESS SUMMARY

"Twenty years from now you will be more disappointed by the things that you didn't do than by the ones you did do."

MARK TWAIN

Principle 1. Determination is the key to all success.

Principle 2. Public speaking can be a powerful tool.

Principle 3. The key to success is differentiation. "Differentiate or Die."

Principle 4. You can only succeed if you try.

Principle 5. If you can find out what people want, you can have anything you want.

Principle 6. It is never as easy as it seems at first.

Principle 7. Always make good on your debt.

Principle 8. Don't expect everyone around you to understand.

Principle 9. To get anything valuable you must swim against the current.

Principle 10. Given the choice it is better to be a big fish.

Principle 11. There must be a place for everything and everything must be in its place.

Principle 12. If you buck the system, you risk the chance of becoming an outcast.

Principle 13. There is always a way to change your circumstances if you are willing to do whatever it takes.

Principle 14. Those who succeed always find the silver lining in every cloud.

Principle 15. Successful business owners learn to do
more in less time.

Principle 16. If you want your message heard you need to start it
with a headline.

Principle 17. If you want to influence a crowd, influence
the influencer.

Principle 18. Sell the benefits, not the features.

Principle 19. When you make them laugh, it lubricates
their wallet.

Principle 20. If you think everyone will be excited about your success, you are wrong.

Principle 21. A successful leader knows the strengths of each individual on the team and leverages it.

Principle 22. A successful practice is framed with a set
of functional systems.

Principle 23. The principle of Have, Do, Be.

Principle 24. Whenever you have the choice, choose affluent neighborhoods.

Principle 25. Word of mouth has always been the most influential
source of marketing.

Principle 26. Treat everyone like the lady of the house.

Principle 27. Know and follow all the laws.

Principle 28. If you want to gather honey, don't kick over
the bee hive.

Principle 29. Investigate the source of your information.

Principle 30. Fear sells better than hope.

Principle 31. Preparation is critical.

Principle 32. Seeing is believing.

Principle 33. It's not how many times you go down that counts.
It is how many times you get up.

Principle 34. You can gather a crowd quicker when you
have an enemy.

Principle 35. One is the worst number in business.

Principle 36. You can learn something from everyone.

Principle 37. If you don't toot your own horn, you may never be heard.

Principle 38. People will pay for what they want.

Principle 39. Collections do not equal profits.

Principle 40. There is power in reciprocity.

Principle 41. You only get one chance to make a good first impression.

Principle 42. Don't confuse busyness with productivity.

Principle 43. Advertising is not optional.

Principle 44. Don't waste your money on plain vanilla advertising.

Principle 45. If they aren't criticizing you, you must be doing something wrong or nothing at all.

Principle 46. Systems create the playing field for winning teams.

Principle 47. Technology can differentiate your practice.

Principle 48. If you are going to butcher the pig, make sure to use the whole thing.

Principle 49. Many successes can be found and borrowed from outside industries.

Principle 50. Make working for you more than a job.

Principle 51. You can't get their money if they can't find you.

Principle 52. A successful model can be duplicated.

Principle 53. No one has ever snuck up on success.

Principle 54. Vision separates the "haves" from the "have nots."

Principle 55. The difference between success and significance is legacy.

Customdentalusa.com or *CustomdentalPartners.com*;
calling ***888.450.9783***
or emailing me at ***Info@CustomDental-USA.com.***
You can also keep up with what we are doing
via *Facebook.*

www.ingramcontent.com/pod-product-compliance
Lightning Source LLC
Chambersburg PA
CBHW052134270326
41930CB00012B/2876